# Personal Renewal

*Also by Letha Hadady*
Asian Health Secrets

# Personal Renewal

*Your Guide to Vitality, Allure, and a Joyful Life Using*
*Healing Herbs, Diet, Movement, and Visualizations*

## Letha Hadady

*Illustrations by Letha Elizabeth Hadady*

HARMONY BOOKS

NEW YORK

Please remember that each person is unique and complex. For that reason you are advised to pay particular attention to your own individual beauty and health issues and to consult with qualified professionals when treating illness with herbal treatments. If you are *currently using medication,* consult with your health professional before altering your program.

The descriptions and identities of persons discussed in this book have been altered to protect their privacy.

Published by Harmony Books, a division of Crown Publishers, Inc., 201 East 50th Street, New York, New York 10022. Member of the Crown Publishing Group.
Random House, Inc. New York, Toronto, London, Sydney, Auckland
www.randomhouse.com
HARMONY and colophon are trademarks of Crown Publishers, Inc.
Printed in the United States of America

Design by Barbara Balch

Library of Congress Cataloging-in-Publication Data
Hadady, Letha.
Personal renewal : your guide to vitality, allure, and a joyful
life using healing herbs, diet, movement, and visualizations / by
Letha Hadady. — 1st ed.    Includes index.
1. Rejuvenation.    2. Health.    3. Mental health.    4. Alternative medicine.
I. Title.
RA776.75.H3 1999
613—dc21                                                          98-28576
ISBN: 0-609-60163-6
10 9 8 7 6 5 4 3 2 1
First Edition

*I was born the product of a Hungarian love song.*
*My parents raised me with love always.*
*My mother showed me the joy of being a beautiful woman.*
*My father made me a perfectionist.*
*I dedicate this book to them, to my wonderful sister*
*and brother, and to all people who wish*
*to learn from their growing pains.*

# List of Illustrations

# Contents

# Part Five: Longevity and Spirit

# Foreword
## by Bernard Jensen, Ph.D.

There is a need for uplift in the lives of people today. The stress that most people live under is unnecessary if we have the awareness of someone like Letha Hadady, who is a blessing to those she touches. Her contribution is not only the advice she has to offer; I feel her book is a treasure of knowledge for the personal self. I felt so good being able to touch the lovely things she has touched. After all, we all need each other for the good we would love to share with each other.

This book is about sharing health ideas. Sharing is something we can use every day, not only for ourselves but for those we meet. This book comes from a heart that is borne into the author's healing work. You feel she is in the right place, giving things to people that they really need. It is very important to realize we must associate with people who are here to help us and add to our lives, rather than those who condemn and destroy.

There is good in everyone, and we must seek that good. It is my pleasure to recommend this book to those who are looking for the higher values in life. There is no doubt that people like Letha are sent to us. They are sent because there is a need for this teaching today more than ever. *Personal Renewal* brings into focus all the things we should be doing from a preventive standpoint. It is so necessary for us to realize how valuable the human body is. It is the application of this knowledge that is most important.

This book will be an asset in keeping you healthy. It will prevent a lot of the trouble we get ourselves into. The worst part of our society today is that we are getting into trouble unknowingly. We need to learn a lifestyle that will bring us the greatest amount of good. We must attract the good in others. You will do this as you take up the values Letha Hadady has expressed in her book *Personal Renewal*.

The prevention of disease is coming in the new day. I believe this book carries us right into that new day, bringing us along to pick up lovely ideas, uplifting help from nature, and ways we can help our family and friends around us. It is for us to be in tune with the cosmos. It is for us to be in tune with the planet. We can know what is on the planet for our good and for our health. We must realize that we have to look at what started our problems and avoid the effects of disease by doing the right things from the beginning. This is a great beginning for those who want a rewarding personal life: I recommend that you start reading this book, *Personal Renewal*.

*Life goes on forever because life is energy——————*

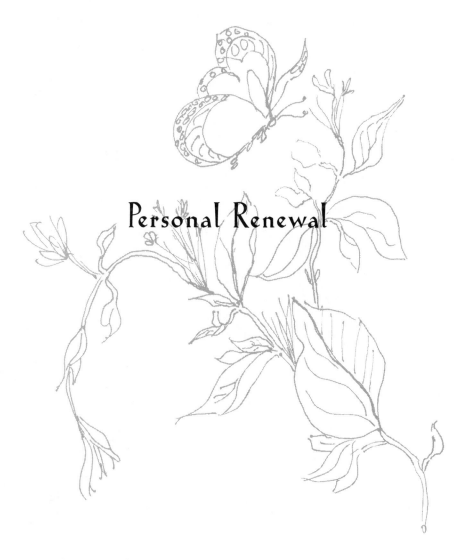

# Personal Renewal

# Introduction

*Suddenly I saw a rainbow . . .*

I grew up barefoot and suntanned in a southwestern town that was spread between the mountains and the valley. When I opened the front door, I could smell evergreens growing on the Sandias thirty miles away. My eyes were filled with sunshine and I walked quietly upon the earth. My desert home protected me like one of its own, a lizard that loves to be lazy. Then one day I took flight.

After attending the University of Paris, I moved to New York. There I studied traditional Chinese acupuncture and herbal medicine and had a professional health practice. That knowledge gave me great freedom of choice: I ignored health fads and medical scare tactics, living as my grandmother and most of her generation had. For years now I have used traditional Asian medicine to prevent and cure illness, pain, and life's shocks for myself and many other people. I have also used it to stay young.

When you work in a private practice at home, there aren't the usual barriers between you and other people that are common in HMOs. No backup crew comes running to assist you in emergencies or to help you with details and paperwork. You base your advice on your own solid training, research, and experience. You speak from the heart and rely on your instincts. At times you may even duel with the angel of death. Many who come to you for help see you as their only hope after spending years and fortunes on medical therapies, which have drained their vitality and spirit. They want a miracle. This allows you to really get to know people.

In the mid-1980s, I began traveling to Asia in order to gather firsthand experience of traditional medicine to share with my clients and students. I lived in tiny villages, visited remote jungles, and witnessed the full impact of Asian medicine in its homeland. I encountered poverty, civil wars, and floods. Crowded trains, poor food, and pollution made travel difficult, but the world of traditional healing that I witnessed was priceless. In Chinese hospitals, whose hallways smelled of urine, I worked alongside doctors who used acupuncture and herbs to cure diseases that are considered incurable in the West. Asia was marvelous, splendid, and shocking. Walking through teeming streets, I would be awed by a glimpse of an exquisite Chinese face but then recoil from the sight of a goiter or a mangled eye.

I became a writer in order to bring the ancient world of healing home and make it American. In my books I talk to people as though they are sitting in front of me. I encourage them to look at, listen to, and understand their vital energy, to see how it influences their mind and heart. Only then can they become their own best healer. Preventing illness and exhaustion requires a greater awareness and dedication than we know. Sometimes we have to become sick before we can make progress in our lives. But I have learned that dealing with imbalance opens many doors.

Books demand a great deal of energy. Writers become crippled while hunched over their computers. They collect fat and wrinkles daily from creating juicy paragraphs while drinking coffee. One of my writer friends calls it an "uglifying" profession. At least I drink pots of green tea to reduce cholesterol and prevent fibroids, and I take handfuls of herbal pills to keep me alert and to prevent poor circulation and indigestion.

Like vast numbers of entrepreneurs who sit for hours on-line, doing business deals by computer, I take vacations with a laptop. I never experienced chronic physical pain until I spent months crunched over my writing, usually with several books in progress. Mornings I awoke with a numb hand and tennis elbow from typing. Hawthorn capsules strengthened my heart and braced my courage. That led to a chapter in this book about using natural remedies to cure computer-related pains such as carpal tunnel syndrome, poor leg circulation, and backaches.

Aging comes from stress, fatigue, and illness, also from disappointment, frustration, envy, hatred, apathy, and bad life choices. Each addiction, divorce, personal loss, or spiritual compromise ages us. I have met young people with black circles under their eyes who were exhausted and old because of cigarette and drug habits begun in their teens. These are not the only addictions: antidepressants and blood pressure drugs often cause weight gain and sexual incapacity. The more we involve ourselves in a magic bullet approach to health—a "this is the only answer for everybody" method—the farther away we get from our innate sense of identity and worth.

To begin personal renewal, you need to reconnect with the positive individual you once were or the person you wish to become. That realization existed during a moment in your life when you felt strong and fully alive, when you realized that anything is possible. I remember awakening early one morning and swimming in the cold waters of the Gulf of Mexico, sunbathing on a pyramid in Oaxaca while watching iguanas, or sitting atop the Dawn Temple in Bangkok. At such moments I felt omnipotent and yet part of the earth.

You may have felt the same surge of power when you hit your first home run or stood on top of a mountain. Inside you a lion roared. Age does not really matter, because energy and vitality generate life force. Improving your vitality can help you to change. You may work in an office or in a profession that takes you traveling, or you may stay home to raise your children: your life can have new meaning when you acknowledge the *original you,* the optimistic source of your inspiration and values.

We may never be able to go home again to childhood, but the original you is inside, tempered and enriched by personal experience. The original you represents your highest ideals and goals. Sometimes optimism requires an act of will. You may say, "I have to look younger, feel stronger, and develop positive habits because my life requires it." However, too often we give up our ideals because we do not have the stamina to carry them through.

Baby boomers—born in the shadow of World War II, who suffered an awkward sexual awakening in the fifties and grew into first marriages, many of which ended like the Vietnam War, in ruin—are beginning to be hit with the problems of aging. By the year 2000 there will be 76 million baby boomers, age thirty-five to fifty-four, controlling over half of America's personal income. Our parents may have accepted rocking chairs or retirement communities, but some of us can remember the promise of the Age of Aquarius. How can we recapture our joyful inspiration?

I explored several alternatives. First, I decided to try one of the most popular current anti-aging therapies: the rejuvenation getaway. Two days later I was eating dates under a Joshua tree in the Mojave desert. I still felt puffy and stiff from sitting at a desk, but I could hear birds singing, and the sweet, warm desert air breathed life into me. I'd flown to a faraway paradise celebrated in movies and song—California. I was writing an article for a health magazine, so I decided to interview a doctor famous for vitamin and hormone therapies, beauty magic bullets that are supposed to take off inches and years. The diet at his spa consisted of raw fruits, vegetables, and inspirational lectures from his staff. I never actually met the doctor.

He represents a widespread trend in gerontology, which defines aging in terms of a reduction of certain hormones naturally produced by the body. This "hormonal shift" approach was originally popularized by the Russians in the sixties, and more recently by books promoting such stuff as melatonin. Fashionable doctors have made their reputations giving patients high doses of synthetic hormones. The drugs' long-term side effects are not well known but may include increased facial hair and acne in women and prostate cancer or heart disease in men. Of course, the hormones can affect estrogen and testosterone levels. It is as though their advocates prefer brief but attractive lives.

After three days of massage, yoga, and walks in the cactus gardens, I felt refreshed. I was offered a treatment said to augment everything from memory to social status. Unfortunately I noticed little improvement. Such treatments are not covered by insurance, and the bill can turn your hair white. There had to be a better way to be rejuvenated. I wanted a program I could do every day at home to improve my beauty and longevity. I wanted a natural way to feel younger and more robust. A magic bullet is more than a popular cure that is supposed to have miraculous results. It is a treatment that works without your participation. Because you are passive, you can become dependent. Most people seek a fast solution to their problems. For that reason, modern laboratory testing, which assumes we will all react the same way to a given substance, is conducive to fads.

I know many practical, natural methods for reversing the effects of aging while improving vitality, sexuality, and looks. Some miraculous anti-aging herbs and foods from Asia are sold in herb shops or can be ordered by mail. Yet others can be found in the supermarket. Back in New York, I searched my herb collection for the appropriate cure for my exhaustion but was overwhelmed by the possibilities. I couldn't move an inch. When you've exhausted physical and spiritual vitality, it is best to heal your heart. When the heart energy is smooth and strong, improvement is possible; you can feel at home in your body and mind.

Mother's place in Albuquerque is an adobe spa, complete with home cooking and mountain views. In desperation I flew home for a week of Hungarian loving and finally began to mend. Everything I know about being a beautiful woman comes from Mother. Her feminine courage, generosity, and sweetness have been an inspiration. After surviving cancer by using a combination of Eastern and Western medicine, she started a new business painting murals. She's in her seventies and always up to something. There's likely to be a painting on an easel in the spare room and brown bread baking in the oven. When I arrived, I found her in the restaurant next door, standing on a ladder, painting a twenty-foot mural of wildflowers. Her wisps of white hair were pulled back with a red kerchief.

Her garden was a profusion of bright color: blue pansies, stately white tulips, pink desert willow, evening primroses, velvety purple irises, yellow forsythia, and poppies. Mornings, we took walks along the Bosque del Apache. Springtime in the Rockies has always been a healing salve to my spirit. These earth elements give me strength—the scent of piñon pine and red clay after a rain, the thrill of sunset over watermelon-colored mountains. A memory shot through me with lightning force. I wanted to celebrate Easter, even though it had passed, with a pilgrimage to a village high in the mountains of northern New Mexico. I drove to Truchas to visit Sabinita, the herbalist.

I love herbal witches all over the world. I have found them in marketplaces and huts from Thailand to Latin America. I follow them into jungles and through deserts and listen, always listen. They speak the oldest language: they whisper of creation as they gather roots and berries to make pills and plasters. They dry leaves and catch lizards. Their hands are old, and their eyes deep from guarding many secrets.

Sabinita is asthmatic and has a limp. Every Sunday she walks ten miles to attend Mass at the *sanctuario*. She'll take a bus a hundred miles to find herbs for her patients. She has cured many illnesses, some say even cancer. I found her in her herb shed, drying snakebroom for arthritis and yerba de zorillo for cramps. She smiled and invited me to stay with her.

The village is so small that when you look over the ridge of the mountain you lose sight of it. Truchas is perched on a rock halfway in space. Days, it's washed with dazzling sun and the color of adobe mud. Evenings, the buzz of crickets mingles with the smell of sage and piñon smoke. A warm breeze blows from the west. It was here that I sat on the edge of a precipice and imagined a rainbow.

If you are wise, you take time to periodically reexamine your life goals. Alone in the mountains, weary from work, far from the city and friends, I wondered, What have I done with my life? Am I satisfied? How can I change things for the better? What in my experience has been truly worthwhile? I touched red-ocher clay at my feet and felt warm sunshine relax my face. I inhaled the fragrance of piñon pine and sage. In that instant I saw, felt, tasted, and blended with the sun-filled energy of the Southwest. I sensed the part of it that had made me. I could begin from there to rebuild my strength.

Throughout my life I have cherished natural medicines made from exotic roots, fungi, seashells, plants, garden herbs, and spices. I have traveled the world seeking wise ancient healing and spiritual traditions. Natural medicines make it possible for you to become young, dynamic, and fruitful because they increase life force. They provide a way for us to become part of the living earth. I offer those rejuvenation miracles to you.

# PART ONE

# THE ORIGINAL SELF

*There is a you that predates all anger, grief, fear, disappointment, apathy, and shame.*

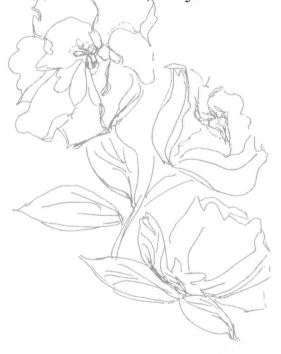

You and I will form an intimate bond as you read this book. I join you as a fellow seeker of inner truth and renewal. We both aspire to beauty and youthfulness and have a commitment to becoming the best we can be. You and I begin and end as friends although we have never met. Reading these words, you may be sitting in your living room, hanging from a subway strap, or relaxing on the beach at Malibu. Our meeting of mind and purpose will allow you to reinvent yourself.

# CHAPTER I

# Choose Your Age

*Renewal is the ultimate makeover.*

This is a demanding book that will give you a second chance. With it you will learn how to take your vitality, beauty, and spiritual wellness into your own hands. You will sense, see, and decide where you are now in terms of your goals and desires for health, then remake yourself based on the insights, pains, and mistakes of the past. From the silence within yourself, the silence at the heart of all creation, you will begin again.

The organization and contents are set up in a unique way to give you as an individual what you need in order to feel fully alive. With the help of my knowledge and experience, you will gain access to a vast body of Asian medicine as it applies to your particular needs. In the process, you will become aware of an array of herbs, foods, and natural products widely used in Asia, which may seem mysterious or miraculous in the West. I suggest mail-order sources for those products in the Herbal Access section at the back of this book, and whenever possible, I recommend easily available natural alternatives from the health food store or the supermarket.

The personalized approach of the treatment programs in this book will enable you to avoid popular fads and scare tactics whether they originate in the excesses of modern medicine or in the misuse of the herbal tradition. Anyone who feels that youth, beauty, and inspiration can be bought in a bottle is a victim of advertising and ignorance.

Rejuvenation means growing younger, turning back the clock. Renewal involves much more. It requires becoming better, making yourself over. It is a positive, active process that must be personalized to be effective. This makeover requires more than a cosmetic or a medical magic bullet or a daily fitness routine. Renewal demands a fundamental understanding of who you are. Now is the perfect time to reclaim your highest qualities and capacities. The insights and experience gained from this process will enable you to suspend your belief in ironclad personal limitations and free you from traps set by parents and teachers. With this book, you can follow your inner guide, using feelings and memories in conjunction with suggested healing herbs and foods, energy-building and hormone-balancing exercises, massage treatments, and visualizations.

Youth and age are partly a matter of habit and training. We have all met wise old children and youthful adults. With my help you can become your preferred age. You will learn to cure chronic pains and fatigue and reduce fat, wrinkles, and hair loss. Eventually you will be able to reverse the results of gravity and prevent the erosion of time because you will have gained energy, vitality, and sexual spark. This process will reveal your fundamental source of inspiration. To accomplish this, you will be asked to look within yourself with love and understanding in order to release old habits.

You may require renewal because of illness, overwork, addictions, disappointments, or self-doubt. My approach is neither a pep talk nor the impersonal data of laboratory studies but is made of earth's highly potent natural resources—herbs and energy—combined with mental exercises that focus on the original you, the person you were before age, exhaustion, worry, grief, and the frustrating world of adulthood hindered you. To shut out such distractions for even a short time allows your loving nature to emerge. It will show you a new path of vitality and spirit.

I developed the rejuvenation programs for this book in conjunction with workshops I've taught for major corporations such as Sony Music Entertainment, the New York Botanical Gardens, and the Staten Island University Hospital. The programs have met with spectacular results. I developed the herbal and diet routines during nearly twenty years of private health practice using alternative medicine in the United States and the Far East.

Asian communities provide compelling information useful for longevity. Japanese people live longer than any other group—unless they migrate to the West. Along with Chinese people, they suffer fewer cancers, fatal heart attacks, and strokes than do Americans. Their diet, lifestyle, and use of traditional herbal medicines are well worth considering. Heart disease and cancer will be discussed in Part Two of this book, as will herbal products originating from Japan, China, and India, which are readily available from American manufacturers and distributors. Using a practical, personalized approach, we can create vigor and the promise of long life.

# How to Use This Book

The aspects of rejuvenation you will stress at any given time will vary depending on your physical and emotional needs. I suggest that you begin by reading Part One. You will learn to create a healing space, a safe place from which to begin your individual program. Each of the subsequent four parts stands alone and can be used separately later, as needed.

Because people have differing levels of time and need for renewal, I've added shortcuts that summarize the chapter at a glance. Chapters begin with a list of goals and materials that enable you to mentally begin working on renewal issues. Most chapters contain a five- or ten-day treatment plan which incorporates that chapter's information in a convenient format. I've included a section called Keys and Links on the last page of most chapters; it is set off by a hummingbird icon for easy location. The keys are distilled recommendations from the chapter, and the links—like computer links connecting websites—relate that chapter to others.

The overall structure of this book is highly personalized, because *you* will decide the best course to follow. You may want to enhance your looks and vitality, balance your mood after an important event or life change, or use an augury such as the *I Ching* to guide your selection of treatments. Use the interactive sections of this book as you like—mark up the questionnaires and tear out pages to post on your wall. Make renewal a gift to yourself.

Unlike my previous book, *Asian Health Secrets,* which was organized by illnesses such as arthritis, colds and flu, and menstrual problems, this book works with the body, mind, and spirit as a whole. You provide the book's structure by choosing the parts you need most. Any discomfort will comprise physical, psychological, or work-related elements. Only you can know which of those you need to work on. What we think of as chronic illnesses are actually arbitrary constructs made by Western medicine. An ancient holistic model—Asian medicine and its alternative American offspring—combines insights on illness prevention and anti-aging together as a guide to better living.

I hope the multifaceted approach presented in this book becomes a daily pleasure. Renewal problem-solving is made more fun with virtual trips to beauty spas and healthy parties. My integrated programs provide opportunities for improving the quality of your diet, exercise, and personal reflection. Renewal reaffirms all that is good about you. It is so powerful that it works even if you are unaware of its immediate benefits.

When you eat an apple, you might not be aware that the apple is simultaneously helping you to prevent cancer and lose weight as it rids your body of impurities. You might not know that the apple is lifting your spirits while it is cleaning your teeth. Eating an apple does many things at once. *Personal Renewal* combines methods and approaches that work together smoothly. Chapter 8 offers a yearly illness- and aging-prevention calendar containing suggestions for weight loss and beauty, which simultaneously build immunity and high energy.

Here is a brief overview of the book that will help you decide which course to follow. The book is organized into five parts. Five is the universal number in Chinese medicine. For ancient sages, the earth was made up of five elements. There were five seasons and five sorts of energy that demanded movement. This book begins and ends with you: if you decide to read through the book consecutively, the movement of your attention will shift first inward to observe yourself in terms of your past and your habits, then outward to redefine your relationship with others.

Part One: The Original Self begins in your healing space. There, with natural remedies and visualizations, you will eventually rediscover the *original you*. That more positive self will be your witness as you gain strength and vitality. It will help you remember who you were and who you want to become. This section of the book may allow you to get in touch with the frustrations, dreams, and fears that lie under the surface of your consciousness, the part of yourself that is hidden in memory. Throughout the book, new directions will arise as you transform outdated personal goals.

Part Two: Damage Control offers ways to recondition your face and hair with natural remedies. I describe ways to prevent and treat illness- and work-related pains, including backache, varicose veins, and carpal tunnel syndrome. You may start to feel your body in a different way after using herbs that stimulate circulation. Freed from chronic pain, you may discover an adventurous side of yourself. You will find that certain foods and herbs that prevent illness also enhance beauty, flexibility, and emotional balance.

Part Three: Eternal YOUth covers ways to get into shape and lose weight safely and effectively. Many of the same herbs prevent diseases aggravated by poor digestion and circulation. We will match certain herbs with exercise for local fat reduction. Special teas used along with massage and essential oils create natural face-lift treatments. We will have a great time losing weight with a virtual trip to Miami Beach for a watermelon and cherry fast.

Part Four: Energy, Vitality, and Sexuality is a playground for personal sparks. This section helps you decide which energy tonics work best for you. You can enhance sensuality with a romantic dinner of aphrodisiac herbs. A hormonal massage increases sexual responsiveness while providing rejuvenating benefits.

Part Five: Longevity and Spirit involves you in healing your broken heart. You will have the chance to withdraw from the world to clarify what you really want from renewal. I will show you how natural herbal and homeopathic products can help you get in touch with your own wealth of feelings and memories and then help guide you to future happiness. Because I've provided the links between related chapters, you can use Personal Renewal as a changing organic whole, a multidimensional approach to creating the person you wish to be.

Health fads come and go with great regularity and too often with dangerous side effects. Anyone who claims to have found one magic pill or one healing method to stop aging for all people is a quack. We are individuals who benefit from self-knowledge. That requires intelligence, compassion, and insight. The experience of an herbal tradition also helps.

Much of what is considered alternative medicine originates from cultures older and wiser than our own. Herbs, homeopathic remedies, and foods become part of us. Often they are absorbed as nourishment, while remaining natural catalysts for change. Throughout the world the herbal tradition is well established, and international research information is available from a variety of sources. I have listed some in the Herbal Access section at the back of this book. I've also included a few major American distributors for easy access to herbal products. In Asia, herbs are most widely used in Chinese medicine, which is practiced in China, Japan, Thailand, and elsewhere. In America, many new health products use Asian herbal ingredients or an Asian eclectic approach to healing.

Unfortunately the herbal tradition remains limited until we can use it most effectively, applying specific herbs to individual problems. I have written this book for people who wish to learn about themselves with the process of renewal. Aging involves complex processes, including genes, hormones, immune system responses, environmental insults, personal habits, and everyday mistakes. We also age mentally, emotionally, and spiritually. Thanks to certain modern medicines, we are living longer than previous generations. At the turn of the century, the average American lived to be forty-seven. Now that age is over seventy. That gives us plenty of time to reflect on the quality of our lives. If we were Taoists, we might silence our yearnings and spend years seeking inner guidance, but this is another world. Today we need skills to help us live joyfully and productively, to create our own unique beauty.

Neither the latest scientific theories and laboratory studies on aging nor rejuvenating magic bullets can accomplish renewal. You must personally protect your youth, beauty, vitality, and intelligence with good habits. Healing herbs, foods, and creative imaging promote confidence and well-being. More than this, you must share the love in your heart to feel young and happy. What good is rejuvenation if we suffer painful or shallow lives? Renewal is a flowering from within.

It is time for a new awakening.

CHAPTER 2

# A Healing Space

*My healing space brings into focus my
personal joy and clarity of purpose.
It contains the aura of the Southwest.*

---

*Your Goal:* **To create a sacred space somewhere in your home in
which to follow healing and beautifying programs. It can be a whole
room or simply a part of a room.**

*Materials:* **Objects, colors, sights, and sounds that evoke peace,
joy, health, and radiance. These may include: wall paint or fabric;
rocks, gems, shells, and plants; photographs, sacred images, incense,
candles, music, or prayers; sunlight, water, or earth. Make sure to
include hope and benevolence.**

---

Whenever I shut my eyes and think of Truchas, I see adobe brown.
I've searched in vain for that color while browsing through paint
samples in New York hardware stores. I finally mixed it myself by adding
pink to terra-cotta. My adobe wall captures the sunlight in my apartment.
I put sangre de Christo and yerba de zorillo from the *curandera* Sabinita's
garden into a Zuni pottery bowl. I placed that on top of a wooden table in
front of my mud-colored wall. Then I lit white candles at either side. This
became my healing space. Now when I light piñon or Tibetan incense
there, I can feel the room widen and the air soften around me as I breathe
deeper. Time moves more slowly in the desert and high mountains. Even
in lower Manhattan, I can withdraw to my desert to rest.

Your healing space will become your access to the original you. My original self is not synonymous with the Southwest, but the desert puts me in touch with it. There I feel close to the thread connecting my previous lives to the present and future. This opens my field of possibilities: in the sunlight and quiet of my desert healing space, I claim what I want of myself and what I wish to become.

Certain people have described a moment in their lives when all things seem to join in perfect harmony, when they feel they are part of nature. It is an experience of pure clarity and calm. Your healing space is the area in your home where you will welcome such vision: it will become a refuge from everyday worry and the noise of the outside world.

# Create Your Healing Space

Decide where in your home your healing space will be. You can use a wall of your apartment, an entire room, or even a tabletop. The size of the space is not as important as the quality of energy you create there. The space must be in a quiet place where you will not be disturbed.

Your healing space will contain the signature of the original you, the person who was (or who could be) vibrant, enthusiastic, and young at heart. To reconnect with the original you, imagine a time and place when you felt your best and were happy and confident. If you can't remember any such time, sit quietly and relax. Taking slow, deep breaths, let your mind wander to a place where you would most like to be. Imagine that place in full detail. Then mentally answer these questions:

Where are you?

What is around you—the ocean; mountains; wide, luscious meadows; the desert?

Imagine the colors, sights, sounds, and fragrances that surround you.

Do you want to be alone there or with people, spirit guides, or animals?

Now take elements from that visualization and add them to your healing space. What colors will you use? Did you think of the ocean? If so,
paint the wall or use a tablecloth the color of your ocean. Add shells or
seaweed or sun-bleached driftwood. Complete the picture with anything
that evokes *your* ocean. Did you see rocks or plants in your vision of the
original you? Re-create that vision as completely as possible. You are making an altar to your higher self.

Can you find music or recorded natural sounds that remind you of
your vision? What incense or aromatherapy would best apply? Will you
have candles? A bowl of tropical fruit or an evergreen? Add photos or
whatever you need to duplicate what you experienced while remembering the original you.

The point is to make a real healing space. It may take a little time and
effort, but you will be able to take refuge there. You may wish to make an
elaborate creation, even hire a construction crew, but do not be tempted.
The space that will best heal you is one that you make yourself.

Eventually you can make a smaller version of your healing space in
your place of work. That way you will be able to withdraw from stress
whenever you need to be refreshed and renewed.

You may wonder what significance the images in your vision might
have in a larger setting. Of course, images you saw and felt when you were
at your happiest and strongest have special meaning for you, but as elements in the natural world they also reflect potent healing energies. For
example, if you imagined water, a river, or an ocean, that is the element
you need to give you peace and comfort. This may be because you grew
up near water or because you need more moisture in your life. Do you
feel refreshed when surrounded by water? You may find that cool, moist
weather also agrees with you.

Do not place any value judgment on what you see in your vision of
the original you. If you feel better being alone, that's what you need to
heal you now. If you feel you need water or seashells, perhaps you will also
benefit from moistening foods and herbs. But that kind of analysis will be
presented later in this book. For now, accept whatever you experience in
your visualization. Consider it a gift.

# The Five Elements and Your Healing Space

Ancient Asian doctor-philosophers saw us as made up of the same elements as nature. For example, Chinese doctors described five elements: fire, earth, metal, water, and wood.

The fire element, located in the heart, keeps us warm and glowing because it enhances circulation. People are said to be fiery if they are emotional. Fire gives us vitality and brilliance. Add a candle to your healing space if you need endurance and courage. It will warm your heart.

The earth element is located in our digestive center. As the earth bears fruit, our earth element makes digestion possible. The fruits of good digestion are adequate energy and blood production, which lead to health and balance. People are said to be grounded, centered, and at home with themselves when their earth element is thriving. In other words, when digestion is comfortable, we feel at ease. You may wish to add a potted plant to your healing space in order to nurture your earth element. In Part Three of this book you will learn about digestive herbs that can strengthen your earth element.

The metal element in our body is located in the lungs, the large intestine, and the skin. The metal element lets us breathe oxygen and exchange the impure for the pure. When the metal element is healthy, we breathe deeply and exhale fully. We can thus eliminate toxins from the body and mind. Our communication with others is smooth when our breath is relaxed and deep. Smoking or overindulging in spicy foods damages the lungs by causing inflammation. The result is often shortness of breath, anxiety, and skin blemishes.

You may wish to add a rock or some crystals to your healing space to help you relax. Breathing calmly and focusing your attention on these objects may help increase your capacity for compassionate interaction with people and the environment. Have you been deeply hurt in the past?

In your healing space you can strive to purify your emotions, to become clear like a crystal or gem.

The water element in our body regulates the ebb and flow of our internal ocean. It commands tides of hormones and body fluids that affect every aspect of life. We are made up mostly of water. Without its soothing influence, we have fever, thirst, irritability, shriveled skin, and unhealthy hair. When young, we are juicy and fresh. There's an old French saying that babies are born out of cabbages. They call their children *petits chous* (little cabbages) because babies are fresh and sweet. In Part Two, we will learn a number of herbal moistening and blood-building remedies to keep our looks young and fresh. In Part Five, we will discover herbs for increasing sexual fluids. For now, place a bowl of water in your healing space as an offering to your water element.

The wood element, situated in the liver and gallbladder, keeps muscles strong and flexible by ensuring the absorption of calcium. A green twig can bend in the wind. When the wood element is healthy we are flexible; we can change our daily routine without becoming anxious. We can also move about free of joint and muscle pain. We are not troubled by headaches, allergies, and bad temper when the wood element is in balance. We can become like strong trees, rooted into the earth and stretching to the sky. We can make plans and carry them out if the wood element thrives, because our mind is balanced, our actions are organized, and our body is strong and steady enough to carry out our desires.

Incense has been used for centuries to evoke prayer. Perfumed temples and churches throughout the world offer refuge to those seeking wisdom and hope. You may wish to add incense to your healing space, not only because of its spiritual significance but also as a means of respecting your wood element. Tibetan incense, which is traditionally made of delicious natural fragrances such as juniper, sandalwood, and herbs, is especially effective in soothing nervous problems—headache, insomnia, and depression.

You can work toward balancing all five elements by having emblems of them in your healing space. To do this, use some personal token that evokes fire, earth, metal, water, and wood.

You may wish to add something completely different to your healing space. Colors, visualizations, and activities can be added. I have an artist friend who has learned to listen to truths revealed by her spirit. On airplanes, with a sense of freedom that comes from flying, Carol gains access to her creative imagining. She describes it as euphoria—the absence of thought. With movement, she is lifted above ordinary life to experience a place in her consciousness that is without limits, a space between heaven and earth where she can create. The bonds that keep her locked in body and mind are slipped. At the end of the flight she may hardly know her whereabouts. She is stunned like a bird that, having flown through a storm, has found sunlight. Something in her has shifted. She has conceived of a painting. It is not an act of will but a gift of grace—a weightless, timeless state of inspiration like levitation.

Yogis have studied for years in an attempt to achieve this lightness of being. Dervishes have spun like tops to create a new awareness. Those of us who have experienced a moment of insight—when all barriers separating us from our environment drop, when we merge with nature, with God, or with another person—know this heightened state. My friend experiences freedom while in an airplane even though she cannot move about freely but is more or less confined to a seat. The quality of her experience is entirely different from the ordinary because her mind's focus and energy circulation are involved. The normal pull of gravity seems less as our center moves upward in meditation. I think her artistic intention leads her to greater possibilities. At such times the heart opens. We have a sense of "Now I can do anything. Everything is possible."

If movement or any other body sensation frees your imagination, use it in your healing space. You can bathe or dance there, for example. But remember that the insights you gain in your healing space will be charged more strongly than ordinary experience because you will be rediscovering and remaking yourself.

Finding the original you can be the best gift you give yourself. It is the fertile field from which springs all change. Eventually your healing space will be *within* you.

# CHAPTER 3

# The Face
# in the Mirror

*A rose by any other name is no longer a rose.*

---

*Your Goal:* **To develop skills in Asian facial diagnosis in order to analyze internal energy and vitality. This chapter gives you an objective approach for achieving a new self-image.**

*Materials:* **Herbal blood cleansers and liver cleansers, including capsules of dandelion; alfalfa; aloe vera gel added to juice; energy tonics like hawthorn, nettle, damiana, or Chinese ginseng; nervines such as Siberian ginseng to reduce the effects of jet lag and stress; and homeopathic remedies such as kali. mur. (potassium chloride), kali. sulph. (potassium sulphate), nat. sulph. (sodium sulphate), silicea (silicic oxide), and ferrum phos. (phosphate of iron), all at 6x strength. For individual conditions, also see the Keys and Links on page 34.**

---

Call a line a wrinkle and it becomes a problem. Call a line the result of low energy or poor circulation and you open a door to prevention and treatment. The face in your mirror is a picture of living energy that breathes and changes. If you have stared at it for a lifetime only to find faults or search for praise, try to see your face in a new way. Who *is* that person in the mirror? It is not the original you but the result of habits and character. Even those can change when you allow it to happen.

It takes special training to become objective about personal appearance. A healer recognizes not only what actually exists but also—given the best possible health and vitality—what could be, a picture of your ideal appearance. Facial diagnosis is nothing more than comparing your present appearance with the potential young and radiant you. This kind of observation is actually more sensitive than other, more scientific, objectivity because it compares the results of your lifestyle with your original aims. Do you look like the loving, vibrantly alive person you want to be?

# Change Your Energy and Change Your Face

This chapter will give you the tools you need to analyze your energy, vitality, and youth by observing your face. After determining which specific areas require improvement, you can begin to implement healing programs that will influence the factors which underlie appearance— detoxification and vitality. I have provided individualized diets and herbs to correct underlying imbalance. Here is the key: change your energy and you change your face. Your face can mirror your highest aspirations and talents. A loving attitude is beautiful to see, but hatred, arrogance, jealousy, and greed freeze grimaces that can last a lifetime. Our goal is not just to be wrinkle-free but to be liberated from our limits.

To observe your face, sit comfortably in your healing space and look carefully at your face in a mirror. The best lighting is indirect sunlight. Try some observations at different times of the day to see the effects of fatigue and stress.

For a moment, observe your face and hair as a whole without noting details. Imagine that you are looking at someone else; then shut your eyes and imagine how you might look if your skin was fresh and clear, if your hair was thick, shiny, and its original color, and if your eyes were clear, moist, and relaxed. That is a picture of youth brought about by eating well and using the right herbs.

Cooling and cleansing foods and herbs clear the skin. Moisturizing, blood-enhancing herbs add luster to complexion and hair. The same sorts of herbs will calm emotions because they reduce excess acid and indigestible wastes while building vitality. In that way, beautifying herbs can help you find peace and mental clarity.

Your imagined youthful face is your ideal, but it can become your goal when you know the necessary diet and life changes you must make to achieve it. Let's observe your face in more detail so that you understand something fundamental: your face is made of living energy and moisture, which can and must change.

# Your Face Shows What's Inside

The following observations will help you determine your optimum rejuvenation regime. Making the appropriate changes in your diet can reverse visible signs of poor digestion, circulation, and vitality. Your face is a picture of your energy and emotions.

How you present yourself to the world is shown in the way you use your energy. Do you move through life in a determined manner or stand back to analyze a situation and then move cautiously? It depends upon circumstances, but you can observe tendencies in your face. You can learn who you are by observing your energy and intention—how you move through life. When you put your best foot forward, which foot is it?

Determine which side of your face is dominant. Most people have irregular bodies, where one side seems stronger. One leg may be longer or one shoulder higher. This affects energy, movement, and eventually facial expression. Poor energy distribution may result in a squint or twitch. An internal weakness may lead to problems such as poor muscle tone or a lackluster complexion. Recognizing your dominant side can sometimes help you select a balancing regime.

Cover one half of your face, then the other side, with a piece of white paper. Notice if one side seems larger, longer, or fatter. Does this difference correspond with strength or weakness in the same side of your body?

Clench your back teeth and look at your front teeth in a mirror. Do the two front teeth on top line up with the two front teeth on the bottom?

Is your bite crooked? If so, does it correspond with tension in your jaw? Do you have more tension in one shoulder than in the other? If so, you may notice that you have a wince or a stiff expression on the corresponding side of your face.

Are there more blemishes, moles, or injuries on one side of your face or body? If you have more irregularities or muscle tension on one side, that may be your dominant side, the side that moves forward to greet the world. Read on to see if you have adequate energy on that side.

## Right-Dominant People

Right-dominant people often express themselves with a dynamic energy. They think and move quickly when making decisions. Traditional Chinese doctors describe this as yang (outgoing, movement, or processing) energy. During conflicts, right-dominant people are likely to be active or aggressive. When their actions, growth, or change is impeded, they become frustrated and angry. Some develop bad dietary habits. A rich diet, addiction, and strong emotions can lead to liver congestion. Signs of this condition include bad breath and a greasy or coppery-colored complexion.

Do you do everything with your right hand?

Are you impatient when things go slowly?

Do you eat irregular meals or a rich diet?

Do you feel discomfort in your right side or your chest?

Do you frequently suffer from headaches, stiff shoulders, sciatica, sinus congestion, arthritis, high blood pressure, excess cholesterol, anxiety-related heart palpitations, insomnia, vision problems, skin blemishes, or allergies?

Do you experience facial twitches or spasms?

Do you have wrinkles, dry skin, or a ruddy appearance?

If so, you will benefit from the cleansing routine beginning on page 54.

Right-dominant types need to purify their liver and reduce excess acid with bitter and pungent cleansing herbs such as dandelion, aloe, and alfalfa in order to ease muscle tension and smooth circulation. Dandelion, which is slightly laxative and diuretic, reduces water retention, skin blemishes, and breast fibroids. Alfalfa is recommended for arthritic stiffness and vitamin deficiency. You might start by taking two dandelion and alfalfa capsules after meals daily, then work up to a dosage that feels comfortable. One-quarter cup of bottled edible aloe vera gel (available from health food stores) added daily to juice or green tea will reduce sour stomach and bad breath.

Right-dominant types and those who suffer from cramps, spasm pains, headaches, allergies, and nervous irritability need to develop balanced movement, strong muscles, and healthy joints and nerves with the above liver- and blood-cleansing herbs. Cleansing and toning the liver and reducing excess acid will help ensure adequate calcium absorption, which will increase physical endurance and patience.

## Left-Dominant People

Right-dominant people tend to act before they think. However, left-dominant people tend to spend so much time gathering information that they hardly move at all. Left-dominant people are sensitive. Some are trapped in reveries about the past, while others use their personal insights and emotions to do their best work. They try to see and feel everything before they move ahead. Their hesitation goes beyond the old category of introvert: left-dominant types try to digest or incorporate their surroundings. Traditional Chinese doctors say that yin—internal organs, blood, body fluids, emotions, and hormones—determine such actions.

Do you express yourself from your depth of feeling?

Is your complexion a bit pale and pasty?

Are you short of breath, anemic, or depressed?

Do you feel spacey if you don't eat often?

Do you have water retention, a spare tire, or bags under the eyes?

Left-dominant people tend to be slower or more methodical than right-dominant individuals, as much from illness and fatigue as from introspection. Soft facial flesh tone and weak muscle tone may be related to poor dietary habits—caffeine, sugar, and unhealthy fats and sweets. If that is the case, you need to strengthen your internal organs, especially the spleen and pancreas, which are involved in sugar and protein metabolism. Your heart is in jeopardy if you eat too many refined sugar products and oily fat foods, because they weaken circulation. To protect muscle tone, you need to substitute healthy fats and sweets for unhealthy ones, and you might take a heart tonic, such as a capsule of hawthorn after meals. The relation between diet and facial tone will become clear as we look at the shape and color of your entire face.

If you have health and beauty issues from both categories—right- and left-dominant—you will benefit from learning more about your energy. Each person is unique. It pays for you to become familiar with individual signs of stress. They may be signs of inflammation (common for right-dominant types) or weakness (common for left-dominant people).

### Inflammatory and excess acid conditions

Does your face always become flushed after you eat spicy foods or drink alcohol? Do you break out in blemishes under stress? This requires cooling, cleansing foods and herbs.

### Weakness

When fatigued, do you get circles under your eyes, facial puffiness, or a sallow complexion? Underlying weakness can become worse because of allergies, pollution, jet lag, or drinking coffee. Certain tonic herbs and foods can correct internal weakness.

# Facial Shapes and Your Energy

Observing facial shapes is a limited sort of analysis. The facial shape is inherited and can be somewhat adjusted with cosmetic surgery. But energy patterns also help maintain a particular shape. When fatigued you may feel that your face sags. Actually, your vitality is sagging. Because circulation as well as blood and collagen production can improve by increasing your intake of oxygen and certain nutrients, improving vitality with diet can eventually change your face.

## The Puffy Face

Does your face seem puffy?

Do you have water bags under your eyes?

Is your tongue pale and large?

Do you have stuffed sinuses or thick mucus congestion?

If so, you likely have deeper energy problems such as fatigue, shortness of breath, and depression. If the facial muscles lack tone and you experience low energy, Chapter 13, Total Energy for Work and Play, will help you overcome your underlying digestive and adrenal weakness.

## The Slender Face

Does your face seem too long and thin?

Do your cheeks sag?

Do you often have allergies or a runny nose?

Are you short of breath when you're tired or after you eat?

If so, you may also experience poor digestion, chronic diarrhea, chronic fatigue, or low immunity to illness. Chronic diarrhea makes you feel washed out. Eventually, weakness affects muscle tone. Yeast problems such as candida, a cause of poor absorption, can aggravate stuffy nose, poor concentration, low vitality, and sagging skin. Chronic low energy and health problems contribute a great deal to our appearance. They are among the imbalances discussed in Chapter 4, Prevent Illness and Discomfort. The natural face-lift treatments in Chapter 11, Defy the Law of Gravity, will increase facial tone as they lift vitality.

# Facial Hue

Observing your facial hue will help you determine the internal origins of the chronic problems mentioned above. We do not observe the pigment coloring but rather the cast or hue of the complexion and the eyes. This type of traditional Asian diagnosis indicates the underlying energy problems. Healthy people do not look off-color. Their complexion is like a healthy baby's. Occasionally because of stress, illness, or other factors, we develop a different facial hue, the look of illness. Do not worry if you do not clearly see the hue. It is a matter of feeling it. You can become sensitive to your internal problems by studying your face during times of stress. Following is a listing of facial hues, their internal origins, and some possible herbal remedies. You can add any of the remedies one at a time between meals for a few days, then notice the benefits to your energy and the changes in your facial hue. If you experience a facial hue like those below for more than a day or two, consult with your health adviser.

## Red, Blotchy, Ruddy, or Purple Cast

This type of complexion indicates poor circulation, inflammation or fever, chest pains, chronic heart trouble, or addictions such as rich diet, cigarettes, alcohol, or stimulants. Treat with cooling, cleansing, and moistening herbs such as dandelion, aloe vera, American ginseng, and anticholesterol herbs as well as those for high blood pressure. (See "Cooling Cleansing Diet" page 54.) After you have followed this diet long enough to improve your facial coloring, your skin tone will also have improved. You may notice that your mood and concentration are better. Stress and irritability are reduced when the body has fewer impurities.

## Yellowish, Coppery, Brownish, or Greenish Cast

Hues such as these suggest poor digestion, nausea, stuck bile from rich diet or parasites, liver disease, or liver-damaging addictions. Are your lips dry and cracked? Is there a deep line in your forehead between your eyes? If so, they will become worse from indigestion, diarrhea, or parasites. You may also be eating too many cold, raw, or non-nourishing foods. You may be blood-deficient. Reconditioning the liver will help prevent indigestion and impurities in the blood. Use liver cleansers such as dandelion and homeopathic kali. mur. 6x and nat. sulph. 6x, described on page 33.

## Grayish, Ashen, or White Cast

When this type of tinge is seen in the entire face, with dark circles around the eyes or a dark shadow around the entire mouth area, profound fatigue, low immunity to illness, severe allergies, or jet lag are often to blame. Smokers have dull, pasty skin because they lack adequate oxygen. If you need more oxygen or if blood production is low from poor absorption or chronic illness, you will often feel tired and depressed. You may also experience menstrual irregularity, low sexual energy, or chronic asthma. These are all signs of adrenal weakness.

Treat a grayish hue with adequate rest and tonifying herbs, including various forms of ginseng. Chinese ginseng lifts energy. Siberian ginseng soothes nervous exhaustion. Nettle, damiana, and other herbs that strengthen adrenal energy are useful.

If your sinuses feel congested or you have asthma with thick mucus and wheezing, you need a diet of anti-phlegm foods and herbs. See the "Anti-phlegm Diet" on page 59. After you've followed that diet long enough to improve breathing, your circulation can improve. You will enjoy higher vitality, and your mood and skin will brighten.

# Observe Your Face in Detail

The drawing on the next page shows areas of the face and their corresponding internal organs. Long ago Asian doctors associated these parts of the face with digestion, breathing, circulation, and elimination.

Blemishes require cleansing foods, herbs, and plenty of water. The best way to reduce the deeper problems that cause blemishes is to alternate the two diets that begin on page 54. The "Cooling Cleansing Diet" is anti-inflammatory to reduce redness, while the "Anti-phlegm Diet" helps dislodge hard-to-remove impurities. Here are specific areas of the face and the internal processes to which they correspond.

The forehead corresponds to the intestines and elimination. If you have blemishes there, you need to reduce fat, rich, and hard-to-digest foods such as red meat, dairy products, oils, nuts, and sweets. For the purposes of rejuvenation as well as prevention of illness, which we will consider later, it is best to eliminate meat, caffeine, alcohol, and stress.

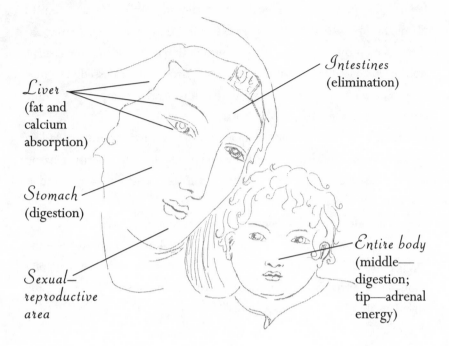

Liver
(fat and
calcium
absorption)

Intestines
(elimination)

Stomach
(digestion)

Entire body
(middle—
digestion;
tip—adrenal
energy)

Sexual—
reproductive
area

The temples correspond with the liver and gallbladder. If digestion is congested by fat or greasy foods, the result is red, angry, or painful blemishes, headaches, and nausea. Avoid peanut butter, fried foods, cow's milk, cheese, egg yolks, and meats.

The cheeks correspond to the liver (on the left side) and lungs (on the right side) and the stomach. If you eat too many hot, spicy foods the entire cheek area will be filled with inflamed blemishes. Avoid peppers, cayenne, garlic, onions, and hot spices.

The nose is associated with the entire body. If the nose looks inflamed or has broken capillaries, the cooling cleansing diet will be most soothing.

The eyes are the mirror of our desire. According to traditional Chinese doctors, the eyes are the outlet of the liver's vitality. The liver produces important enzymes involved in calcium absorption. Therefore a healthy liver ensures strong muscles and good eyesight. Traditional Chinese doctors believe that the liver also contains our soul. Thinking clearly and making and carrying out our plans with care indicate a healthy liver that contains a peaceful soul. Our vision will be normal and our aims in life and interactions with other people will be normal.

A wide blank stare is associated with mental problems or violence. A new occupation has arisen among acting teachers hired to train psychopathic killers to act normal in court. They teach their violent clients to blink instead of stare into space or, worse, at the jury. Of course, not all people who stare are violent. But I'd rather know who might be.

Bulging eyes can indicate thyroid and associated energy problems. Cloudy vision shows poor blood circulation. Bloodshot eyes indicate inflammation that is increased with spicy foods. In all of the above cases, the cooling cleansing diet will improve eye moisture and comfort. In addition, in many cases peace of mind is easier to achieve by eating a cooling, cleansing diet. Start to think of anger as a toxin. As your body becomes less acidic from a cleansing diet, you will relax and your eyes will look less red and cloudy.

The mouth and chin show a picture of the lower body and sexual area. A dry and cracked mouth can result from chronic diarrhea, blood deficiency, and weakness. Blemishes on the chin often appear with PMS because of hormonal activity. If blemishes on the chin appear frequently or if you often experience menstrual discomfort, inflammatory problems or congestion may be affecting your ovaries or uterus. Use both cleansing diets beginning on page 54, alternating them during the month. To avoid sharp inflammatory pain, bad breath, constipation, and red blemishes at PMS time, eat only cooling foods and herbs.

# Your Face and the Original You

There is a connection between the face you see in your mirror and the original you, although it may not be what you think. Your physical appearance can vary drastically from lifetime to lifetime. It will even vary quite a bit in one single lifetime. Is the essential you—the original you—a dramatic brunette, a sunny blond, a fiery redhead, or a cool raven-haired beauty? The outward appearance can change. The elements that remain essential are the aspects of your appearance that come from deep within. Your face is the reflection of your inner being, an image of the quality of your feelings. That is related to your karma. Let's observe it.

In your healing space, imagine yourself alone in a quiet spot. In front of you and at some distance is a forest with trees reaching toward a blue sky. Between you and the forest is a small lake bordered by fruit trees. On the other side of the lake is a group of people and animals who are sick, dirty, poor, and suffering. Imagine each of them in great detail. Listen to what they tell you, and observe what they show you. Imagine in detail the things you actually say and do to help them. Then look into your mirror. The face you see reflects a quality of the original you.

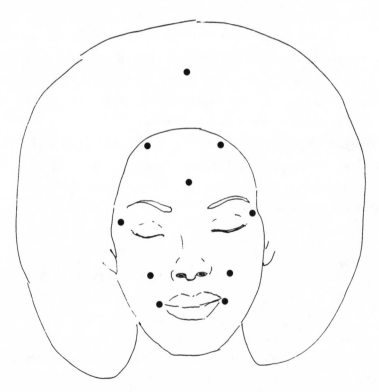

**Place a drop of essential lavender oil here to enliven your tired face.**

# Your Five-Day Treatment Plan for a New and Beautiful You

I have outlined a ten-day treatment plan on page 73 for rejuvenation of the skin and hair, but you can get a head start by deep-cleansing and fortifying your cells with several homeopathic minerals. Homeopathic medicines are made by diluting a trace of something in a neutral base such as milk or alcohol. The advantage in using a homeopathic remedy is that your body absorbs it immediately. If you have arthritis or are lactose intolerant, find a brand of homeopathic medicine that uses alcohol or another neutral substance as a base.

The following homeopathic tissue salts will prepare your body for any of the healing routines in this book because the combination oxygenates the blood and facilitates cell reproduction. After adding these valuable minerals to your diet for only five days, you will see a marked improvement in your skin texture and tone and in your complexion in general: you will notice the glow of oxygen in your face.

For five consecutive days or for up to one month, alternately take the first group of remedies to cleanse your body and the second group to build up your resistance and strength.

## Group one

Take one dose each of homeopathic kali. mur. 6x, kali. sulph. 6x, and nat. sulph. 6x—all taken together. These two forms of potassium and one form of sodium speed up cellular reproduction and cleansing while eliminating excess water retention in the body. They help break down fat and thick impurities such as mucus. The standard dosage will be on the bottle. Wait one hour and then take one dose of the second group.

## Group two

Take one dose each of homeopathic silicea 6x and ferrum phosphate 6x. Silicea gives strength to skin, bones, hair, and fingernails. Ferrum phosphate (homeopathic iron) delivers oxygen to the cells.

Alternate between the two groups throughout the day until you have taken each group five times. Avoid taking homeopathic remedies at mealtime, and wait twenty minutes after drinking coffee.

An easy way to alternate the doses is to add larger doses—for example, ten pills of each separate remedy in the group—to two separate quart bottles of spring water. You end up with one quart of water that cleanses and another that supplies iron and silicea. Gently turn the bottle upside down to mix the ingredients before each use. Each swallow of water equals one cleansing or building treatment. This saves money and supplies needed water to help flush out impurities.

# Keys

Blemishes: dandelion, honeysuckle, burdock, page 62
Wrinkles: astragalus and jujube date, page 181
Mucus discharge: barley soup, radish, homeopathic kali. sulph. 6x
Bruises and injuries: homeopathic arnica 30c

Links: At this point in the book you are free to choose whichever program best suits your personal needs. If you wish to continue refining the beauty of your skin and hair, turn to Chapters 5, 8 (Spring and Autumn), 11, and 12. Otherwise, turn to whichever part of the book suits your interests.

Part Two concerns reversing damage done by overwork, illness, and medical intervention. It offers a year-round prevention calendar.

Part Three offers more help for beauty-energy problems, including weight loss, sagging energy, and menopausal changes.

Part Four will help you acquire energy, vitality, and sexual abundance. In Chapter 15 you will meet a few of my exceptional friends who have learned to strive for and make it to the top while remaining youthful, productive, and mentally and physically flexible.

Part Five allows you to soothe emotional hurts and guides you to find solace in tranquillity and nature.

# PART TWO

# DAMAGE CONTROL

*Overcome fear by using it to your advantage.*

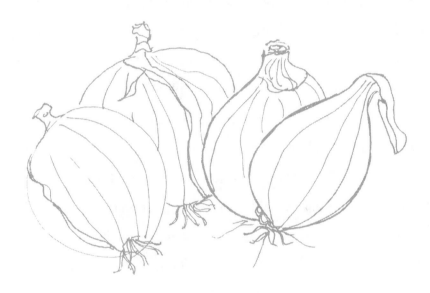

# The Onion and You

Peeling a big white onion makes tears come to your eyes. The pungent odor stays for a moment on your hands. This inconvenient food tastes wonderful when cooked or eaten raw. The water that comes to your eyes cleanses them. The fumes that you sniff while peeling an onion open your breathing. Eating onions helps eliminate cholesterol and eases painful congestion at the joints. Onions help prevent heart trouble and arthritis. Onions are worth the trouble.

Although they require effort on your part, the healing exercises and herbal regimes in the following chapters are also worth the effort. They clear away old karma and life's debris, the signs of aging and illness. Healing experiences need not be disagreeable. You can clear your senses very well by drinking a cup of delicious Chinese chrysanthemum tea (page 63), and you can remove a layer of dead skin by using a skin brush (page 140). The pleasure of rejuvenation comes from finding what works best for you.

# CHAPTER 4

# Prevent Illness and Discomfort

*To be or not to be: that is the question.*

*Your Goal:* **To determine your energy type in order to prevent illness and aging with individualized remedies that are in tune with the season.**

*Materials:* **Cleansing herbs including aloe vera, myrrh, and dandelion; anti-inflammatory foods including cumin, coriander, fennel seeds, celery, red cabbage, and rice or oat milk; stimulant herbs such as hawthorn, green tea, grape-seed extract capsules, ginger-and-mint digestive tea; and mixed trace minerals and vitamins.**

The best health care is always sensitive to individual needs. Still, you may wonder, Do I dare to take personal responsibility for my well-being? How can I avoid the sea of troubles resulting from prescription drug dependence or the slings and arrows of outrageous medical bills? Can I use medical testing and advice as tools for greater understanding rather than as the final answer? It comes down to this question: Do I dare to claim my body as my own?

The benefits of prevention far outweigh the consequences of merely doing nothing. Fear is aging. The fear of illness is doubly aging because it reinforces itself—the more you fear it, the sicker you become. To avoid falling into an anxious torpor, you must take active steps toward prevention.

*Personal Renewal* is more than a resource book for rejuvenation. It is my herbal confession, in which I share some of my favorite nostrums for the discomforts of illness and aging. Unlike most people who work and play hard while looking over their shoulder and waiting for disease to strike, I eliminate fear with prevention.

Our goal is the educated prevention of illness and aging without sacrificing pleasure. In the yearlong rejuvenation calendar beginning on page 105 I emphasize diet. However, I also recommend movement, chiropractic adjustments, massage, mineral water spa treatments, and anything else that increases your joy, well-being, and vitality.

Enhancing digestion and breathing gives the body more energy. One sure way to help both is by eating simple wholesome foods. I have been forced to become healthy. I've lived a high-pressure, mass-media, big-city life, and I have traveled extensively in remote areas. Like most travelers, I have come down with various jungle maladies. This means that I cannot digest rich foods such as meats, cow dairy products, and sugary sweets. So much the better for my energy and cellulite! In addition, I boost my energy while reducing cholesterol and fat by drinking pots of green tea daily. For indigestion, I add fennel seeds, mint, or catnip to green tea. Homeopathic carbo veg. 30c (vegetable charcoal) settles the stomach and eliminates bloating and indigestion. Here is a brief summary of my approach.

At appropriate times of the year I prevent fibroids, heart trouble, arthritis, and exhaustion rather than fear them. Prevention is fairly normal for health-minded people. The difference is that, given my lifestyle, I expect to get sick, so I actively take steps toward *treating* the malady by taking a smaller dose of the natural cure. From spring through autumn, I normally prevent tumors and joint aches by taking cleansing Asian herbs appropriate for cancer and arthritis. During autumn and winter, I treat exhaustion and depression with blood-building and energy tonic herbs. I try to step up my cleansing routine during parts of the year when I need it the most and I can best feel the results. I usually take along Chinese anti-tumor herbs when we vacation in Vermont or Palm Springs, where the environment is cleaner and I feel less stress.

Anti-fibroid herbs such as a combination of one-quarter cup of aloe vera gel taken daily in juice along with two capsules of myrrh can reduce impurities, including fat and excess acid from the body. By stepping up my cleansing routine, my disease-prevention plan becomes a beauty–weight loss program. I enjoy the cleansing process. Herbs heighten my senses as they speed metabolism. By using cleansing herbs regularly, I can relax and forget about disease.

## Prevention and the Seasons

Atmospheric conditions can affect cleansing. Springtime humidity and pollen cause problems in circulation and water retention, which lead to joint pain, headaches, and allergies. Spring and autumn weather increase discomfort from excess acid conditions and mucus congestion. If I didn't use refreshing herbs and spices including cumin, coriander, and fennel before and during those seasons, I might suffer intense pain and lethargy.

The dry chill of autumn and winter sedates vitality and breathing. That's why many people suffer from skin problems, asthma, fatigue, and depression when days grow shorter. My autumn healing routine contains pungent foods such as radishes, onions, ginger, and bitter greens, which prevent these problems.

The trouble with most illness prevention plans is not that they don't work—it's that they are boring. Few people are willing to commit themselves to a frugal diet for the rest of their lives. They may eat fruits and vegetables for a week or a month before they binge on a loaf of bread, a chocolate cake, or some other bad habit. Deprivation intensifies desire. However, using a variety of remedies that are in tune with the season makes our quest for youth easy and fun. We reap the benefits of becoming part of nature.

## How to Proceed

First, determine your best schedule for rejuvenation. I might take several weeks of cleansing herbs when pollen fills the air. But you may not have the time. Try to be regular with the rejuvenation practices I describe even if only for one day a week. If you need to lose weight, turn to page 141. I have included many prevention herbs in the diets in Chapter 9, Let's Get into Shape.

Do the activities that I recommend at a time of day when you can focus on what you're doing. Send out some sort of "do not disturb" signal to friends and family. This would be ideal. But in reality, I've gotten used to swallowing handfuls of herb pills on the run, and I still feel as if I'm eating a salad.

If you consult a chiropractor, massage therapist, or other health expert, try to incorporate what you've learned into your rejuvenation routine. I've outlined my own plan, but please adjust it to suit your needs. Be generous—give yourself enough time to make changes, while encouraging your body, mind, and spirit to renew themselves.

## Organize Your Fear and You Will Conquer It

When we worry about possible illness or panic to the point of total denial, we cannot prevent it. I prevent the illnesses that are most likely to affect me, those increased by stress, pollution, and age; those I may have inherited; and those related to my energy type. However, I don't prevent all of them at once but fit them into my yearly schedule.

One way to determine possible discomforts is by analyzing your energy type. I presented useful keys to that sort of analysis in *Asian Health Secrets: The Complete Guide to Asian Herbal Medicine* (Three Rivers Press, 1998). Here are some additional pointers to guide you in determining the illnesses you are most likely to get.

## The Five Elements and You

We and all living things are made up of the same elements. Ancient healing traditions have named them fire, earth, metal, water, and wood.

The nature of these elements determines our circulation, metabolism, breathing, elimination, and reproduction as well as our mental and spiritual makeup. Although we each have all these elements, one or more will be significant for us. One will be more sensitive or will play a bigger part in our lives. Here's a brief description of each energy type. Do you see yourself in them? Under stress your reactions may vary, but you will tend to react in certain predictable ways, according to your energy type.

# The Fire Person

*Signs:* Flushed complexion, easily excited

*Imbalances:* Anxiety, insomnia, mania, giggle or fast chatter, heart trouble, hysteria

Fire people have a natural sensitivity to stimuli such as caffeine, overwork, acidic foods, and hot spices. They suffer from chronic fever illnesses, high emotions, anxiety, irregular heartbeat, chest pain, or depression. They can be devastated by rejection.

When fire types have high blood pressure or emotional upset, they feel flushed or hysterical. They can get carried away with fantasy or ambition without touching ground. They live in their heart center, romantic life, or art for art's sake. Sometimes they fear that they cannot feel anything without feeling pain, so they push themselves and other people to extremes. Fire types require calming and, occasionally, total retreat from everything in order to regroup or brood.

They need to ease heart action by avoiding unhealthy cholesterol and fat in their diet. They may have to lose weight in order to reduce stress. They require balanced relationships and work that engages their high ideals and love of humanity. They may wish to save the world, but unfortunately they may lack the focus, clarity, or endurance necessary to do their work. In that case certain tonic herbs will help fire people to fulfill their dreams.

Chinese herbal remedies that facilitate memory, increase mental clarity, and prevent insomnia such as Ding Xin Wan can be very helpful for fire people or for anyone suffering from extreme stress, hardening of the arteries, irregular heartbeat, or chest pain. Directions are in English. Like most Chinese patent remedies, Ding Xin Wan can be ordered from the sources listed at the back of this book. Another herb useful for high cholesterol, overweight, and lethargy with slow heartbeat is hawthorn. It tones the heart muscle, making its action stronger and smoother. Anyone under extreme stress who has a weak heart can take one capsule after meals.

## The fire person and prevention

Fire people or those with chest pain or emotional discomfort should prevent anxiety, fever, heart trouble, insomnia, and overweight during the entire year. Intemperate climate, "hot" emotions, stimulants, and extreme fatigue are harmful. See the reference to Raw Tienchi Ginseng powder on page 240.

# The Earth Person

*Signs:* Spare tire, bon vivant, sweet tooth, sugar blues
*Imbalances:* Diabetes, hypoglycemia, overweight, ulcers,
worry, obsession, addictions, mood swings

Earth people have a sweet tooth and often suffer from indigestion or feel empty in their center. They demand rich foods and congenial gatherings. They can be excellent cooks or people who constantly digest their work, mulling over a problem for hours. They may gorge on sweets for lack of love or spit out relationships when they become "fed up." They may suffer from excess acid, burning ulcer pain, faulty digestion, and excess weight. They crave sweets, bread, pasta, and other carbohydrates, especially when they are tired or depressed, which is rather often. They get spacey when they do not eat regularly and when they overindulge in sweets.

Those with ulcers or diabetes require cooling, moistening herbs such as asparagus, aloe, and spices such as fennel and cumin. For hypoglycemia (low blood sugar), they require herbs such as ginger and mint to stimulate digestive acids and enzymes.

Earth people fear not having enough of something. It might be food, money, happiness, friends, or some other necessity. They love plenty of everything and crave comfort and security. Unlike fire people, who become unbalanced by excitement and insomnia, earth people can become so attached to their routine, home, job, or loved ones that they lose sight of the prize or even of themselves. They become stuck in the soup, unable to change.

Earth types may want to eat up your time and energy. Others might give of themselves until they are empty. They need to balance their blood sugar and their need to consume or act out. They need to give and take, not just one or the other but both.

Digestive remedies are extremely helpful for earth types for maintaining steady, predictable energy and harmonious relationships.

## The earth person and prevention

Earth people and those with junk-food addictions should pay particular attention to diet in spring and autumn, avoiding sweet, creamy, and oily foods. Barley, ginger, radishes, and other pungent or diuretic foods will help reduce congestion leading to pain, lethargy, and depression. For bad breath or indigestion with burning pain, add bottled aloe gel to tea or juice daily.

# The Metal Person

*Signs:* Long nose, arms, legs, and fingers; breathy voice

*Imbalances:* Addictions, asthma, depression, fatigue, sallow complexion or blemishes, seclusion, morbidity

Metal people are sensitive to cold, dry air. They catch colds and flu frequently and run from drafts and air conditioning. Weak metal types suffer from chronic diarrhea or shortness of breath. Some metal people feel vulnerable and weak from lack of oxygen. They often make matters worse by smoking. Metal people suffer from all sorts of addictions and depression, especially during autumn.

Metal people may crave hot spices, rich creamy foods, or difficult relationships, all of which impair their energy. They tend to drive themselves with solo work or be content to stay home alone. Their ideals or perfectionism make it hard for them to work with others. They can become an angel of hope and inspiration when their work involves helping others. Making decisions and new situations make metal types feel vulnerable. Such things require energy. They may feel overcome with grief after the loss of a loved one or a collapse of self-esteem. They strive to control people or situations with precision and elegance.

When metal people fall into addiction or despair, they withdraw, fabricating a hostile world from which to escape. They fear closeness and the influence of others because social interaction requires energy, concentration, and, ultimately, oxygen. They need to expand their sphere of activity by increasing their capacity for smooth, deep breathing.

Certain asthma and energy tonics will help metal people feel stronger and more confident. They ought to avoid foods that cause congestion—all dairy products, red meat, white flour, fried foods, and gooey sweets. A cooling diet featuring oats, barley, rice milk, and vegetables, including leafy greens, celery, okra, onions, and red cabbage, will help protect metal people (and others) from inflammatory rheumatoid arthritis.

## The metal person and prevention

Metal people are wise to protect their stamina during autumn and winter with pungent herbs and foods that reduce phlegm congestion. A cup of cinnamon-ginger tea keeps colds away.

# The Water Person

*Signs:* Grayish or ruddy complexion, puffy or dark circles
   under eyes
*Imbalances:* Water retention, obesity, menstrual irregularity,
   sexual dysfunction, low immunity to illness, anxiety,
   depression, greed, paranoia.

Water people crave salt, cola drinks, and foods with low nutritional value. They are sensitive to cold, humid weather, fatigue, pollution, and noise. Most things tire water types. One Chinese doctor said that water people live and suffer a long time. They sometimes have a low reserve of vitality brought about by chronic illness and long-term hassles. Despite this, they frequently exhaust themselves either out of self-interest or for the sake of others. When water types overwork, they have so little vitality left that they can only sit and consume books, chocolates, or television programs. They do not have enough mental clarity or physical stamina to be selective but take life as it falls into their lap.

Water types may suffer from global overweight, heart trouble, chest pain, kidney problems, chronic infections, and inertia. Their sexual energy and drive can temporarily soar, then drop very low. When their energy is used up, they become all desire and no strength. When run-down, they are subject to chronic illnesses such as fibroids, diabetes, chronic fatigue, and other major threats, including cancer. Having little stamina, they can become extreme and fearful. Water types fear a lack of recognition (annihilation), which can turn them into control freaks. When inspired, they can move mountains. When self-indulgent, they become mountains. Deep down, they sense they cannot protect themselves. Water types frequently become paranoid about illness and death. Courage requires energy, which they lack.

## The water person and prevention

Water people or those who have worked too hard or who frequently have jet lag, infections, or addictions to medical or street drugs need to protect their vitality with nutritional and herbal remedies. Because of cold weather and diminished light, autumn and winter are important times to protect adrenal energy. You know your adrenal glands need help if your lower back aches, you have urination problems, and you feel wiped out.

Resistance becomes low when we are depressed and fatigued. Some medical researchers have proven that T cells decrease temporarily after a big emotional shock. If we build up our adrenal strength, we have not only more energy but also more emotional slack to deal with stress. Herbal adrenal energy tonics will help water people year-round, as will slimming herbs. Energy-boosting slimming teas are convenient, but weight loss herbs must be taken only after water people are strong enough to lose weight. Wholesome low-fat, easy-to-digest foods, mixed trace minerals, homeopathic gold, and lots of vitamin C can help the water person retain stamina.

Preventing high cholesterol and fibroids with herbs is wise for water types. This can be done at any time during the year for a month or more at a time (see page 131 for details on cancer prevention). Water people and anyone suffering from chronic illness should alternate cleansing herbs with building herbs in order to protect energy.

# The Wood Person

*Signs:* Angular face, muscular body, nervous, high-strung
*Imbalances:* Headache, arthritis, allergies, spasms, anger,
jealousy, frustration, arrogance, intolerance

Wood people are subject to spasm pain and allergies because their liver is sensitive to excess acid, alcohol, spice, or oily foods. The wind or stimulants can irritate their nerves. They may become out of sorts when they do not get their way or if anyone tries to tell them how to do something. Often hard-driving and well organized, a wood type might be a department head, an athlete, an artist, or a businessperson. They thrive on competition and play to win. When "liverish" and jaundiced, they pout, yell, get a spasm, or can't decide on anything.

They crave many foods, but when their liver is acting up, they crave alcohol, fats, fried foods, and sweets, which harm their circulation and mood. Digestion is weakened by poorly digested fat, which encourages jaundice, nervousness, headache, sciatica, and bad temper.

When their arthritic stiffness or headache feels hot, wood persons benefit from cooling, cleansing herbs such as aloe vera, which reduce acid. Dandelion helps reduce constipation, fibroids, and gallstones.

Wood people fear aging because they have so many projects and passions that they want to have time for them all. They need to develop patience with others and with themselves. They also need to refresh their body and mind with cleansing green plants. Chlorophyll builds blood, nerves, and muscles. Certain headache or insomnia remedies, such as valerian, a nerve sedative, are helpful to ease stress.

## The wood person and prevention

Spring is the season when the wood person, or anyone addicted to hot spices, liquor, or fatty and oily foods, needs to cleanse the liver with bitter and pungent green foods such as dandelion, burdock, skullcap, and watercress. Weak persons who are subject to chills or allergies also need to build resistance in the fall.

# Elements in Combination

You don't have to be a wood person to have wood problems. That goes for all five types. Anyone can become unbalanced due to stress, pollution, emotional upset, or any number of other reasons. Your weakness will be reflected in your energy type. You will intuitively sense which element is vulnerable at a given time. These symptoms can also help you decide.

*Fire:* Irregular heartbeat, panic, stutter, poor mental clarity
*Earth:* Hunger, acid regurgitation, nausea, indigestion, mania
*Metal:* Asthma, fatigue, skin rashes, depression
*Water:* Fatigue, low resistance, poor sexual energy, backache
*Wood:* Jaundice, nausea, allergies, rage, trembling

# The Elements and the Seasons

According to traditional Chinese medicine, the five elements correspond to certain seasons. During the associated season, the element is most vulnerable and most active. For example, in spring we expect wood element problems to surface more frequently. The timing may vary slightly in your area, but the seasons roughly correspond to the following:

*Fire:* Summer or hot weather
*Earth:* Indian Summer or humid weather
*Metal:* Autumn or dry, cold weather
*Water:* Winter or cold, damp weather
*Wood:* Spring or windy, polluted air and allergy season

You will be wise to prevent problems before they occur by following my recommendations for those seasons. Chapter 8 provides a yearly schedule to organize your rejuvenation around the problems that naturally occur each season. You will be able to modify the calendar to suit your needs, adding information from later chapters.

# Five-Day Prevention Plans

The following programs will get you started in the right direction to prevent major health problems associated with the five elements. Choose whichever plan suits your present needs regardless of your energy type. We all suffer from the same sorts of stress at various times. To cure existing illness, you will need to follow the specific healing routines described throughout the book for a longer period of time, but you will quickly achieve positive results with these programs. You can purchase Asian herbal ingredients from mail-order sources listed in the Herbal Access section.

## Fire: Excess Cholesterol and Circulation Problems

Take large daily doses of antioxidants, including vitamins C, E, B$_3$ (niacin or niacinamide), B$_6$, folic acid, and liquid extract or capsules of grape seed *(Vitis vinifera),* along with five to ten cups of Chinese or Japanese green tea daily. If you don't like the taste of green tea, add mint or try taking six green tea capsules daily. Add lots more fresh fruits, vegetables, and seeds to your diet. Give yourself a daily massage such as the one on page 283. Take a fifteen-minute walk daily and increase it to a half hour or more. Consider taking a dance class or one in wine tasting. Fewer people have heart trouble in France's red wine regions.

## Earth: Ulcers, Indigestion

For ulcers add daily doses of vitamin U. Eat raw cabbage, or drink cabbage juice. Add a pinch of cumin powder to hot teas. Avoid hot spices, alcohol, and coffee. See other ulcer remedies on page 209.

For bloating and indigestion, drink ginger tea. Slice a piece of raw ginger one inch square by one-quarter inch thick, add hot water, and steep for five minutes. Add a sprig of fresh mint, lemon grass, or a few fennel seeds or star anise. Also useful is catnip tea. Don't argue with anyone during meals. Take a walk after you eat.

## Metal: Shortness of Breath, Thirst

Add more oxygen to your body by increasing iron and potassium. See page 62 for directions on using homeopathic kali. sulph. 6x and ferrum phos. 6x. The added oxygen will give you more energy and ease your breathing. Reduce excess thirst by drinking American ginseng tea or chewing slices of the raw root. Homeopathic pulsatilla 30c reduces excess mucus congestion and related depression.

## Water: Fatigue, Sexual Weakness, Poor Memory

Vitamin C, zinc, calcium, magnesium and mixed trace minerals, and handfuls of gotu kola capsules daily will reduce stress. Nettle and damiana capsules or tea will help build adrenal vitality. Take a dosage that works for you; six to ten capsules of each daily may be required. Nettle is especially useful to reduce allergies. Damiana is reputed to improve sexual strength when taken over a period of several months.

## Wood: Joint Aches, Headaches, and Nervousness

Avoid hot spices in general and cold, raw food or drinks first thing in the morning. Daily drink one-quarter to one-half cup of aloe vera gel in apple juice while taking one to four capsules of myrrh. If your aches are very inflammatory—with burning pain, red-colored skin, dark-stained discharges, and angry feelings—use less myrrh. Take a warm bath, light Tibetan incense, and listen to music to relax. Massage your feet and rub them with oil, adding pure essential sandalwood or jasmine. Skullcap tea or capsules will help you sleep and cure liverish headaches.

# Free Radicals, Rejuvenation, and the Five Elements

One major current anti-aging trend concerns free radicals—charged free-floating particles that are strongly attracted to other substances such as polyunsaturated fats in cell membranes and certain cellular proteins. Free radicals set up damaging internal chain reactions associated with illnesses such as heart disease and cancer. Antioxidants are the good guys that help destroy free radicals. We used to think that vitamin C and E were the best antioxidants until researchers started looking into why French people have fewer heart attacks than Americans even though they eat everything slathered with cream, butter, foie gras, and cheese. The latest theory is that red wine, red grapes, and grape seeds are chock full of antioxidants. Grapes are also an excellent source of bioflavanoids, which makes them potent rejuvenators.

I always wanted to live like Heidi, with a kindly older man in the Alps. We'd herd goats and make red wine from our own vines. When I looked in New York for the health food store version of grape-seed extract in capsules, I found them to be so expensive that I decided to live my dream. Here are two recipes for Letha's Grape-Seed Wine. Since I make an herbal extract, which requires three weeks of brewing, I normally use brandy or vodka instead of wine.

Start with a bottle of quality brandy. You may prefer vodka because it is a higher proof and more neutral tasting for a stronger extract. Buy a pound of red grapes from the supermarket. To wash the grapes, bring the entire pound—fruit, seeds, stems, and all—to a simmer in spring water. Pour off the water and place the grapes, with their seeds and a couple of inches of the vine sliced in small pieces, in your blender. The berberine found in wild grapevine and root has been used traditionally to cure headaches and liver inflammation. Besides, the vine gives the wine a tart flavor. Blend the grapes, seeds, and stem until they turn liquid; then pour the mixture into the liquor and store this brew, in airtight bottles or decanters, undisturbed in a cool, dark corner of your kitchen for three weeks. After that time—voilà!—you can serve the grape-seed extract, twenty drops per dose, in a glass of red wine.

A variation of this recipe may be necessary if you cannot find grapes with seeds; we have managed to engineer fruit, leaving out the best part. Empty thirty grape-seed extract capsules into a quart of liquor (try rum, vodka, or gin, for starters) and steep it for three weeks. One quart of grape-seed liquor will last longer and taste better than the capsules. This heady brew works well for all seasons and all five elements.

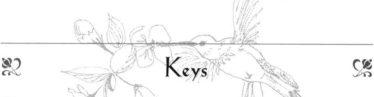

# Keys

*Fire*—homeopathic ferrum phos., kali. phos.
> Heart trouble and high cholesterol: hawthorn, celery, carrot, green tea, Chinese Tuo Cha tea
> Panic: homeopathic aconite 30c
> Fear of upcoming events: homeopathic gelsemium 30c

*Earth*—zinc
> Ulcers: aloe, cumin, cabbage
> Weak digestion: ginger
> Diarrhea with weakness and shallow breath: gentian extract

*Metal*—homeopathic kali. sulph.
> Mucus: radish
> Dry cough and thirst: American ginseng
> Weepy sadness and excess mucus: homeopathic pulsatilla 30c

*Water*—homeopathic nat. mur., homeopathic gold, vitamin C
> Exhaustion with pale tongue: clove (see ashwagandha, page 111)
> Exhaustion with red tongue: see fo-ti, page 226, and Shilajit, page 244

*Wood*—manganese, homeopathic nat. sulph.

Spasms and cramps: aloe

Anger: aloe in the nose (see Lung Tan Xie Gan Wan, page 216)

Bilious liverish headache with nausea: homeopathic nat. sulph. 30c or nux. vomica 30c

Allergic swelling, swollen throat and allergic asthma: homeopathic apis. mel. 30c

## Links: Also see Chapters 6, 7, 8, 12, 13, 16

# CHAPTER 5

# Rejuvenate Your Complexion and Hair

*Beauty emanates from life force and generosity of spirit.*

*Your Goal:* To use two basic diet programs to rebuild and recondition your complexion, hair, and fingernails.

*Materials* (for two diets):

Cooling, cleansing foods and herbs—Teas: green tea, catnip, mint, cilantro, burdock, nettle, dandelion, gotu kola, fennel seeds, aloe vera, and natural sweeteners, including Herba Oldenlandia Diffusa Beverage, available from Chinese herb shops. Grains: oats and white rice. Herbs: parsley, mint, tarragon, celery seed, cumin, dill, coriander, or fennel seeds. Vegetables: spinach, squash, watercress, cucumber, and asparagus. Fruits: berries, cherries, dark grapes, lemon, mango, melons, apples. Homeopathic remedies: belladonna 6x, ferrum phos. 6x, and arnica 6x.

Anti-phlegm foods and herbs—Roasted chicory coffee substitute, adding cardamom, ginger, clove, anise, or cinnamon. Grains: barley and corn. Vegetables: carrots, celery, scallions, beets, peas, broccoli, white potatoes, and horseradish. Fruits: pineapple, papaya, and fresh strawberries. Also see special Asian herbs for acne, dry skin, irregular pigmentation and broken capillaries, thinning hair, and bloodshot eyes.

A flawless face that cannot show love is a death mask. With herbal potions valued for generations, we can improve an internal reservoir of beauty to promote the growth of new skin, hair, and fingernails, the outward signs of our blood.

The following programs—the cooling cleansing diet and the antiphlegm diet—enhance beauty because they remove impurities from the blood while improving circulation and breathing. This makes more oxygen available to rejuvenate the cells. These diets can be made part of your overall health and wellness routine or used as a remedy after dietary excesses. I've included several skin and scalp treatments you can make in your kitchen. You can order the recommended Chinese herbs by telephone, fax, or e-mail, using the addresses in the Herbal Access section.

# Cooling Cleansing Diet

F*or red dry tongue; inflamed blemishes and dry skin; bloodshot eyes; flaky scalp and dull hair with split ends; and bad breath.*

This is a very practical diet that reduces indigestion, constipation, cramps, and irritability. Blemishes, ruddy complexion, and broken capillaries are signs of chronic inflammation, poor elimination, and stress caused by liver congestion, spicy or fried foods, alcohol, caffeine, cigarettes, hormone irregularities associated with menopause, chronic fever conditions, exposure to pollution and harmful chemicals, emotional upheaval, or other factors.

The following teas and foods reduce acid conditions that lead to poor complexion with dry, itchy, or blotchy skin and scalp, liver spots, bruises, bloodshot eyes, thinning hair, bad breath, and fragile fingernails. If these are long-term problems for you, make sure to add some cooling foods to your daily menu. You should also remember that excess acid exacerbates other inflammatory conditions such as arthritis, allergies, certain cancers, chronic bad temper, and hot flashes.

# Cleansing Teas

Cleansing herbal teas that are slightly bitter, laxative, and diuretic purify the body while they help repair jangled nerves. Drink as many cups of the following teas as you wish per day: green tea, catnip, mint, cilantro (a tea that increases urination), burdock, nettle, dandelion, or gotu kola tea. All but gotu kola are slightly laxative. *Important note: Avoid laxative herbs during pregnancy.*

Nettle has been found to be particularly helpful for pollen and fur allergies. You can make a strong tea, using one tablespoon of spring nettles per teapot, or take six to ten nettle capsules daily. If you like the taste of coffee but suffer from its enervating effects, try brewing a substitute made from roasted chicory or dandelion root. Simmer one teaspoon to one tablespoon dried herb per cup water.

## Sweeteners

Herba Oldenlandia Diffusa Beverage (Sheshecao Instant Beverage) is a Chinese herbal product available in Chinese stores or by mail order from sources listed in the Herbal Access section at the back of this book. It looks and tastes like raw sugar crystals but contains valuable cleansing herbs that clear the skin. Superior Sheshecao Beverage, made from the same beautifying herbs, adds powdered pearl. A substitute for this might be sugarcane juice or maple syrup to which you have added ten drops of skullcap liquid extract.

Fennel seeds are also a sweetener that can be brewed as tea or chewed dried all day. They are digestive and slightly laxative.

It is best to avoid sugar and honey because they are irritating. Honey is congesting when heated. That means it turns into an indigestible glue.

# Bitter and Cleansing Herbal Teas

Bitter is better for cleansing whenever acidic impurities are involved—when blemishes are red, irritated, and swollen or when eyes are dry and bloodshot.

Aloe is a solace for rough, irritated body and mind. It is given by angels to the desert so that you can smear it on external burns and scars and drink it to heal ulcers, menstrual cramps, constipation, and angry blemished skin. The aloe plant is extremely healing and alkaline, containing large amounts of vitamin E. Its laxative and diuretic action reduces excess acid. Aloe is the best plant to treat temporary bad breath from acid indigestion or nervousness. You can drink the gel straight from the bottle you buy in a health food store— many people like the fresh, clean taste—or you can add it to apple juice.

If you don't mind drinking a tea that makes your mouth pucker, add up to one-quarter cup of aloe vera juice or gel and one-eighth teaspoon of turmeric powder per pot of green tea. Take one capsule of myrrh, a natural antibiotic, with each cup.

You might also add the following cleansing herbs to green tea: catnip, mint, dandelion, burdock, cilantro, or gotu kola. Catnip and green tea are especially soothing for ulcers or colic. This can show up on the skin as redness and irritation near the mouth. Dandelion and burdock are especially useful for reducing red blemishes that appear during PMS. Cilantro, the leaf of the coriander plant, is useful for puffy face and body during PMS or other times. Gotu kola is a nerve tonic useful for anxiety, fatigue, insomnia, poor memory and concentration, and nervous skin rashes, especially those that are increased by sugar and excess acid, such as herpes. Use it daily if you are under stress.

## Cooling Grains and Cooking Herbs

The best cooling cleansing grains are those that help the body retain important moisture while they cleanse excess acid. They include cooked oats and white rice. Enjoy them along with your hot cleansing tea from the above list. Season cooked grains with cooling herbs like parsley, mint, tarragon, celery seed, cumin, dill, coriander, or fennel seed.

## Green Vegetables

All greens are laxative and nourishing. They contain valuable vitamins and minerals that will help prevent serious problems related to poor calcium absorption. Greens improve your eyesight, muscle strength, and flexibility as they clear your skin. The chlorophyll contained in green vegetables is basic to radiant good health. Greens also build blood and bones.

For a quick lift, steam spinach and whip it in a blender with water, adding protein powder or soaked peeled almonds.

Green squash is cooling and laxative. Watercress, raw or cooked, makes beautiful skin. Try a meal of greens or add liquid chlorophyll to a cup of water and drink it before bed to build blood and clear the skin overnight.

## Cooling Fruits

The following fruits can be eaten raw or whipped into spring water to make a refreshing drink: berries, cherries, dark grapes, lemons, mangoes, melons, and apples. Do not mix fruits with grains or vegetables.

### Almond Milk Bedtime Beauty Drink

This recipe can be adapted to suit individual needs. If you need more calcium because of arthritis or constipation due to weak muscle tone, add a supplement.

> ¼ cup peeled almonds
> 1½ to 2 cups rice, soy, or goat's milk
> 1 pinch turmeric powder

Soak the almonds all day in spring water. Discard the water. Whip the soaked almonds in the milk until blended. Add the turmeric, and (optional) sweeten with Herba Oldenlandia Diffusa Beverage. Drink this warm at bedtime.

Almonds are an excellent source of protein and calcium. These milks are not congesting like cow's milk. Goat's milk contains natural sodium, which helps calcium absorption. This drink nourishes and clears the skin because turmeric is antibiotic.

## A Pleasure Cure

In case you feel deprived when eating cleansing diets and herbs, I have provided some pleasure cures. This tasty one-step apple pie takes minutes to prepare. Use it as a dessert or main dish to clear skin blemishes.

### Apple-Fennel Pie

**4 crisp red apples**
**1 tablespoon dried fennel seeds**
**1 teaspoon dried tarragon**
**2 tablespoons Chinese Sheshecao Instant**
   **Beverage powder**
**Juice of ½ lemon**

Quarter the apples and blend them, along with all of the remaining ingredients, into a chunky paste in a food processor. Then fold the blended ingredients into a prepared pie shell, cover with foil, and bake at 400°F. for 45 minutes or until soft. Serve this pie cold or it will be too fragile to cut.

As a variation, I am likely to blend a block of raw tofu into almost any pie recipe. The tofu adds richness, making the pie a main dish. It also helps hold the pie together. If you have digestive problems, add cardamom or mint powder or pumpkin pie spice.

## Cooling Diet: A Sample Menu

### Breakfast
Hot green tea with aloe and peppermint
Cooked oatmeal with raisins and optional Herba Oldenlandia Diffusa (Sheshecao) sweetener (or maple syrup substitute) and oat milk

### Lunch
Green salad with fresh herbs
Vegetable crepes with lemon or cranberry sauce or sushi with hijiki seaweed
Green tea

### Dinner
Pasta with pesto or fresh vegetables and olive oil (avoid garlic and onions)
Mixed raw vegetable salad
Cooked bitter vegetables (squash, celery, or endive)
Red wine or green tea

*Between meals*
Aloe with five dandelion and alfalfa pills twice daily
Supplements: calcium and magnesium, mixed trace minerals
with 50 mg zinc, 50 mg vitamin B6, vegetarian formula vitamins
A and D
*Before bed*
Almond milk or a piece of sweet, ripe fruit

---

# Anti-Phlegm Diet

For thickly coated tongue; dull lifeless skin color and tone; dark circles and bags under eyes; thick mucus discharge from sinuses, eyes, and blemishes; water retention or puffy face; or greasy, oozing sores.

These anti-phlegm foods and herbs are an excellent addition for anyone who needs more oxygen because of smoking or asthma. The spices clear white, runny mucus. If the discharge is yellow, green, or infected, use the cooling spices (cumin, coriander, fennel, mint, dill, and parsley) listed above. If a thick discharge continues, you may require additional antibiotic herbs.

Use the anti-phlegm diet during spring and autumn or during a spell of humid weather. It is a reducing diet because it aids metabolism. That makes it useful for sinus congestion, premenstrual bloating, and depression. By speeding metabolism and adding oxygen to the body, it helps heal oozing, watery, or itchy blemishes.

## Digestive Teas

To green, oolong, or mint tea or to roasted chicory coffee substitute add one or more of the following digestive spices: cardamom, ginger, clove, anise, bay leaf, or cinnamon. Drink the tea hot or at least without ice to ensure smooth digestion.

## Cleansing Grains

Grains that clear congestion such as barley and corn are drying. Flavor barley soup with any of the pungent spices listed above. I like to roast big red peppers stuffed with cooked barley and chopped carrots, celery, scallions, ginger, parsley, and mint. You may wish to add other pungent spices.

## Pungent Vegetables

No anti-phlegm meal is complete without radishes. You can cut them into your cucumber salad, eat them raw or cooked. Large white daikons are recommended to reduce congestion, but any other type of radish will do. Other anti-phlegm salad vegetables include carrots, peppers, onions, cauliflower, spinach, endive, beets and beet greens, peas, broccoli, white potatoes, asparagus, Brussels sprouts, cucumbers, and watercress.

## Two Anti-Phlegm Fruits

Papaya and pineapple contain enzymes that speed digestion and reduce congestion. Add these delicious fruits to cooked foods or eat them raw as a snack. I've heard of a successful treatment for chronic asthma and low energy consisting of raw pineapple and hot green tea first thing in the morning. It makes a great summer breakfast. Soak dried fruits to remove the high natural sugar content. Raw pineapple is so digestive it may burn your tongue.

## An Anti-Phlegm Bedtime Drink

The vitamins and minerals in this drink will build strength and improve breathing. That will help prevent indigestion, insomnia, and blemishes.

### Spinach Zest Drink

**¼ pound raw spinach or watercress**
**1 slice of raw ginger, ¼ inch thick**
**⅛ teaspoon or less of prepared horseradish**
**Juice of 1 lemon**
**Turmeric powder**

Steam the spinach or watercress along with the ginger slice in spring water until it turns dark green. Remove the ginger and add the lemon juice. Blend until smooth and drink warm with a dash of turmeric powder.

# A Pleasure Cure

If you want to really enjoy ridding yourself of congestion, add this delicious drink to your diet. One meal of this each day will improve your breathing. Added oxygen will increase vitality while it clears your skin. I enjoy this digestive drink after the gym or as a summer breakfast.

## Pineapple Protein Drink

**1 tablespoon vegetable protein powder**
**1½ cups raw pineapple or juice**
**½ cup water**
**Fresh strawberries**

Blend one tablespoon of mixed vegetable or egg-white protein powder into 1½ cups pineapple juice and ½ cup water. Or whip in a blender the protein powder along with 1 cup raw pineapple and ½ cup water. Top with fresh strawberries.

---

# Anti-Phlegm Diet: A Sample Menu

## Breakfast
Hot green tea with a dash of turmeric, ginger, or cardamom
Rye toast with cranberry sauce
Dry cereal with rice milk

## Lunch
Mixed vegetable salad with radishes
Barley soup with carrots, celery, parsley, and scallions
*or*
Fresh pineapple and sprout bread
Oolong tea with ginger or clove

## Dinner
Steamed vegetables, including corn, squash, potatoes, and carrots
*or*
Borscht with blinis and applesauce (no cow dairy products)

## Between meals
Dried fruit or anti-phlegm vegetables, dulce seaweed or dried sunflower seeds, clove tea (for wheezing and exhaustion)

Calcium with mixed trace minerals, laxative and diuretic herbs
as needed, and five pills each of papaya and alfalfa twice daily

*Before bed*

A cup of hot tea made from fresh ginger, clove, dried orange
peel, and mint leaves

# Herbal Treatments for Special Problems

## Acne and Eczema

The following tea recipe contains one blood cleansing herb and one
antibiotic herb to help clear and heal the skin. Simmer one handful each
of dandelion herb and honeysuckle flowers in a liter of spring water. Strain
the tea and drink one to three cups, hot or cold, a day. Excess use of these
and other cleansing herbs can lead to diarrhea. Avoid them if you are pregnant. Make sure to take acidophilus daily.

Another treatment for acne is a combination of several homeopathic tissue salts. They are readily available in British, European, and Latin American
pharmacies and in American health food stores. Add one dose each of homeopathic kali. mur., kali. sulph., calc. sulph., and silicea, all 6x strength, to
one liter of spring water. Sip one-half cup three times daily. Alternate drinking this blend with another one made with homeopathic iron: add one dose
of homeopathic ferrum phos. to a liter of spring water. Drink from the two
mineralized waters daily to cleanse and build skin luster and clarity. The
combination of the two adds needed oxygen to the body.

The dosage can be as often as you like, usually three teacups of each
mixture alternating throughout the day. When using homeopathic remedies wait one half hour after eating, drinking coffee, or brushing your teeth.

## Antibiotic Skin Cleansing Pills

When skin blemishes are long-term or include carbuncles—hard
encapsulated pustules—use a combination of blood-purifying antibiotic
herbs such as Lien Chiao Pai Tu Pien, a Chinese herbal formula available
by mail order. (See the Herbal Access section.)

The dosage is most often four pills twice daily. It can be combined with other cleansing pills such as capsules of the herb oldenlandia diffusa (sheshecao). The ratio is for every four pills of Lien Chiao Pai Tu Pien, take two capsules of sheshecao.

A possible substitute for the Chinese patent remedies is a combination of herbs that are anti-inflammatory laxatives, antibiotics, and skin cleansers including burdock, dandelion, skullcap, echinacea, and cascara sagrada. Do not use echinacea for more than two days without adding acidophilus to balance intestinal flora.

Warts fall off after taking homeopathic thuja 200c five times daily for three to six months.

## Sinus Congestion and Facial Beauty

Stuffed sinuses can make you feel and look uncomfortable because they decrease your breathing. Difficult breathing reduces needed oxygen. Eventually the skin loses its luster. For a five-day treatment plan that reduces underlying mucus congestion conditions, turn to page 33 at the end of Chapter 3. Here are some more allergy-reducing herbs that will improve both your energy and your looks.

Pollen Allergy Pills are available by mail order from Chinese herb shops listed in the Herbal Access section. Such remedies contain herbs that clear phlegm and increase local circulation affecting the face. Directions for dosages are in English inside the box.

Two herbs often used in Chinese sinus allergy pills are magnolia buds and Chinese white chrysanthemum flowers. If you have a garden you may wish to grow them yourself. Simmer a handful of each in two cups of spring water for no longer than five minutes. Strain this and drink a cup warm at least one-half hour after meals.

Many homeopathic combination remedies used to clear sinus congestion also treat discomforts such as headaches, thick mucus that drains into the back of the throat, and a face stuffed with painful congestion. Homeopathic remedies frequently used are combinations such as hydrastis can. 2x, calcarea carb. 3x, and kali. bichrom. 3x, made by Washington Homeopathic Products in Bethesda, Maryland.

# Dry Skin and Premature Gray Hair

Chapter 12, No Fear of Fifty, covers these problems in detail, offering a variety of natural remedies. Fo-ti (in Latin: *Polygonum multi.*; in Chinese: he shou wu) builds blood and moisture to overcome these symptoms of dryness and deficiency. Fo-ti comes in capsules and is available in health food stores. The Chinese form also comes in pills called Shou Wu Pien or as a semisweet liquid, Shou Wu Chih. (See the Herbal Pronunciation Guide and the mail-order sources for patent remedies in the Herbal Access section.)

Adjust the dosage as needed. Start with one health food store fo-ti capsule or five Chinese pills between meals three times daily. Pay attention to how it affects your breathing and digestion. This moistening herb should be taken between meals because it is not digestive. It increases phlegm congestion for people with poor digestion. Avoid it altogether if you have a cold. If it makes you feel sleepy or congested, add digestive herbs such as ginger or Chinese ginseng.

Famous Chinese longevity elixirs such as Thousand Year Spring Tonic contain those two celebrated herbs, shou wu and ginseng, along with royal jelly, an excellent source of B vitamins.

You may enjoy making your own beautifying tonic by adding nourishing fruits, herbs, and spices to brandy or sweet vermouth. Start with a cup of red grapes because the skin and seeds are rich sources of antioxidants and bioflavonoids. You can add crushed red grapes and seeds, along with any of the following berries, which are high in vitamin C and iron: raspberries, strawberries, bing cherries, prunes, or peaches. For flavor, add a few star anise, a cinnamon stick, and some dried orange peel. Steep this brew in a wine bottle at room temperature for three weeks so you have a zesty healing tincture.

# Thinning Hair

Hair loss that is related to blood deficiency becomes worse with stress. You will also see dry skin, bloodshot eyes, and a ruddy appearance. Cooling, moistening herbs and foods such as those found in the Cooling

Cleansing Diet are very helpful. Also make sure that you get daily doses of 1,000 to 3,000 mg lecithin, 3 to 6 grams of vitamin C and 400 I.U. of vitamin E. Niacin or niacinamide frees microcirculation in tiny blood vessels, bringing more blood to all extremities. So does six capsules daily of ginkgo. This protects the hair at the roots and shafts like an invigorating massage. Add daily doses of homeopathic iron, ferrum phos. 6x, and homeopathic potassium, kali. sulph. 6x, in order to help oxygenate and heal dry, flaky scalp.

A popular Chinese capsule remedy, Shang Fa, contains blood-building herbs combined with those that enhance circulation in the head. Dosage instructions are in English, but should vary with your needs. If moistening, blood-building herbs are sedating, take them on an empty stomach before bed.

Here is an alternate remedy loosely based on the Chinese one. Its ingredients are eclipta, yellow dock, and homeopathic silicea 6x. Eclipta prostrata is used for blood and moisture deficiency affecting the liver, bone marrow, bones, skin, and hair. Yellow dock provides iron and enhances blood and lymph cleansing and circulation. Homeopathic silicea heals the hair, skin, and bones while ridding the body of impurities. The combination facilitates a deep cleansing and revitalizing movement of energy from the blood outward to the hair.

Using addresses listed in the Herbal Access section of this book, you can order powdered eclipta from bulk herb companies or from Chinese herb shops, where it is called han lian cao. Fill empty capsules from a health food store, and take three capsules or one teaspoon of the powder twice daily. With each dose of eclipta take three yellow dock capsules. Throughout the day take five doses of homeopathic silicea 6x to treat chronic weakness.

To reverse the underlying inflammatory condition associated with blood-deficiency hair loss, add cooling foods and herbs such as those in the anti-inflammatory diet found on page 54. A cooling, moistening diet and the above herbs will leave your skin, eyes, and hair sparkling in a matter of weeks.

## Scalp Massage to Stimulate Hair Growth

Healthy hair is sometimes unable to surface because the scalp is clogged with dry skin. A massage using pungent herbs and cleansing oils helps the skin breathe and the hair grow. A number of excellent hair tonics, moisturizers, and shampoos are sold in health food stores. One of my favorite companies is African Formula Products in Gainesville, Florida. They use more healing herbs and oils in their products than I can list—with no harsh chemicals or animal testing. Their Bio Pure leave-on conditioner and moisturizer has herbs, oils, shea butter, vitamins A and D, and vegetable protein from soy and wheat to nourish and groom the hair.

If you want to make an invigorating scalp massage to use at home, you can add essential oils and herbal extracts to safflower oil. If your hair and scalp are dry and scaly or if you have dandruff, use equal parts of aloe vera gel and jojoba oil instead of safflower oil. The important herbal extracts to include are nettle, comfrey, horsetail, tea tree, and calendula. They soothe and lubricate the scalp and stimulate hair growth. Choose several essential oils from among lavender, rosemary, cedar, peppermint, sandalwood, juniper, honeysuckle, jasmine, or rose. Be gentle when massaging your scalp and leave in the mixture overnight.

## Quick-Fix Treatments for Tired, Bloodshot Eyes

Your eyes will feel relaxed and moist if you enhance the blood circulation surrounding them. To do this, dip a Q-Tip in aloe vera gel and gently clean the inside of your nose. Then add extra gel inside your nose for a while. The cooling gel will relax the nerves leading to your stressed brain. As head circulation improves, you will feel cooler and your eyes will have increased lubrication. If your sinuses are congested, add one drop of tea tree oil to the aloe vera.

To reduce eye puffiness and help prevent glaucoma, I recommend Bilberry Complex made by Sundown Vitamins in Boca Raton, Florida. Also eat or brew along with tea a handful of wolfberries, also called fructus lychii, lycium fruit, fruit of the matrimony vine, or gou jee tse in

Chinese herb shops. They are tasty little sour-sweet dried red berries that build blood, but they are laxative when used to excess.

In Chinatown several varieties of Ng Far Char tea, a combination of loose herbs, are sold. The major ingredients are prunella and Chinese chrysanthemum flowers, both of which clear the sinus area and cool the eyes. You can mix your own brew combining herbs that treat fever and inflammation from the eye and sinus areas. Here is my favorite sweet-tasting herbal tea used to clear vision and comfort the eyes.

### Letha's Sparkling Eyes Tea

**1 handful *Prunella vulg.* (xia ku cao)**
**1 handful Chinese chrysanthemum flowers**
   **(ju hwa)**
**1 handful Chinese dried red rose buds**
**Essence of Tienchi Flower Instant Beverage**
   **(sugar substitute)**

This is a mild, sweet tea that cools and refreshes the skin and eyes. If sinuses are very congested because of allergies or hay fever, add a handful of dried magnolia buds.

Add all the ingredients to a quart of cold water and bring it to a boil. Simmer for 1 minute and let it cool slightly before drinking. Enjoy this brew between meals as an afternoon or evening tea. It is best not to drink this tea during the same day as the combination of eclipta, yellow dock, and homeopathic silicea (page 65), or you may feel too scattered and cooled out.

# Wrinkles

In Chapter 11, Defy the Law of Gravity, I tell you how to turn the following Chinese herbal formula into a delicious skin-firming liquor. Persons allergic to alcohol will prefer this prepared as a tea: simmer a handful each of Chinese huang qi (astragalus), dang shen (codonopsis), and dried red jujube dates (*Ziziphus jujubae;* in Chinese, da zao or hong zao) in a liter of spring water for about one-half hour.

Drink this pleasant, delicately sweet tea throughout the day between meals only. It slows digestion by bringing moisture (and digestive acid!) to the skin by increasing sweating. The dosage is up to four cups daily.

# Blotchy Skin or Irregular Pigmentation

Skin becomes discolored or freckled for a number of reasons. If it is not hereditary but related to aging, pregnancy, menopause, endocrine irregularity, liver disease, or poor diet, herbs can reduce or eventually reverse it. More than likely, if you got age spots after forty or from taking birth control pills, the condition was related to liver congestion. Wearing a hat or sunscreen will not help, but the following herbs will.

Yunnan Universal Herbal Products Company in China makes a liver tonic with the unlikely name of Fairily-Kit Facial Pigmentation Remover. This is not a skin-peeling remedy. The misnomer arose because the Chinese refer to moles and other such discolorations as "extra skin." These green-and-white capsules do not remove skin; they contain valuable blood-building herbs as well as several to increase circulation such as millettia, atractylodes, and tang kuei. The dosage is one or two capsules twice daily.

Facial Pigmentation Remover is less moistening than a related Chinese formula called Patch Removing Pill. The latter is recommended with a dosage that does not exceed three bottles because its blood-building herbs might become too moistening for some people. Taking too many moistening herbs could slow digestion and increase sinus congestion or head cold symptoms such as nasal stuffiness and low energy. That can be reversed by taking the remedy along with digestive herbs such as ginger tea.

The advantage of taking a Chinese tonic remedy instead of having a dermatologist zap off moles is that herbs get to the root of the matter. Moles can come back or increase in size and number but internal factors such as hormone imbalances can be adjusted with herbs. The advantage in taking blood-building remedies is a reconditioned liver, the benefits of which include calmer nerves, improved vision, softer, prettier skin, and less chance of menopausal concerns.

# Fragile or Broken Capillaries

People have poked fun at my "blue blood." The offspring of Hungarian cousins from an old noble family, I have nearly transparent skin that makes my veins visible. It's not a problem except when I have to color-coordinate my clothes with my blood vessels.

On the other hand, many people complain about broken capillaries, called spider veins, which look like tiny red or purple lines or a pinkish wash on the face, arms, or legs. These are not inherited from intermarriage of noble families but are influenced by hormones, stress, spicy foods, hot emotions, and energy imbalances.

Treating spider veins gives a fabulous income to quite a number of dermatologists, laser-zapping and electric needle–wielding plastic surgeons, and beauty cream manufacturers, but nothing works without certain risks. Electric needles and lasers can leave permanent scars. Saline fluid injections, usually done for spider veins on the legs, can discolor the skin. Facial massage and moisturizing creams do no more than soothe the skin surface, ignoring the deeper area where the problem lies.

I once took my tiny spider veins to a large, curly-haired uptown New York dermatologist. A friend of Woody Allen, he proudly showed me stills from movies he had appeared in. Dr. Actor kindly explained that I needed the latest up-to-the-minute, extremely expensive laser to treat the capillaries he could hardly see around my mouth. Last year's laser was outdated.

Somewhat chagrined, I took what he called my nearly invisible capillaries to Chinatown. There the problem was treated with a shrug. Chinese women have different skin. They look ageless. They may also be less concerned than obsessive blond blue-bloods. I decided to try some things myself.

Coptis-Evodia Tablets, manufactured by Seven Forests and ordered from Chinese herbal distributors, is recommended for acid stomach, belching, and hypertension. It also cools dry red skin at the mouth and cheeks because of anti-inflammatory liver-cleansing ingredients. Three times daily, combine three pills with a dose of a cooling antiseptic skin formula such as Lien Chiao Pai Tu Pien (or its substitute described on page 63), and it works even better. Either Chinese herbal combination reduces facial redness and inflammation. Neither alone is enough to prevent broken capillaries.

A daily drink made from Chinese Po Nee Tea combined in a teapot with a handful of dried Chinese rosebuds and sweetened with Essence of Tienchi Flowers instant drink is a refreshing way to tone facial circulation and reduce redness. Essence of Tienchi Flowers is instant sugarlike granules that reduce hypertension, irritability, insomnia, "pimples around the mouth," and grinding your teeth in your sleep. It may save dental as well as dermatology bills. I find this drink too sweet by itself. It has a cloying taste and is best used as a sugar substitute.

For people who prefer using homeopathic remedies, the best alternative treatments would correspond to the energetic functions of the above herbs—in other words, they would increase blood oxygen in the cells and stimulate surface microcirculation of the skin. These would include anti-inflammatory homeopathic remedies for red blotches and fiery capillaries such as homeopathic belladonna 6x and ferrum phos. 6x. Arnica montana 6x increases circulation for bruises and discoloration. Kali. sulph. 6x, sulphur 6x, and silicea 6x treat chronic skin conditions.

Acupuncture also works well for reducing facial redness and swelling, especially considering that such problems often have an internal origin. Acupuncture points frequently used for treating the face are located in the arms, hands, and feet because they bring down inflammation. Other points used include those that treat the heart and circulation; they are located on the feet and the solar plexus. (See page 171.)

I use a small Swiss-made cold laser instead of needles when doing acupuncture. After a few treatments, using points on the chest, stomach, hands, and feet, the acupuncture was successful: the facial redness and circulation improved. My capillaries became even more invisible.

# Skin Treatments for External Use

The best home remedies are the easiest to make and use. Here is a peek at my own cleansing and moisturizing routine. I use ingredients that are safe enough to eat.

## Moisturize and Protect

To moisturize and protect the face, scalp, and body, I mix a few drops of jojoba oil and aloe gel in my hand, then rub the mixture on after a bath. Expensive superfatted creams clog the pores and feel greasy. For variety, you can blend your favorite essential oil into the jojoba-aloe mixture. I enjoy essential cucumber oil for its lovely cooling fragrance. You might like to juice raw potato and cucumber and add them to the aloe and jojoba oil. Because of their high potassium content, the vegetables cool and tone the skin.

## Increase Facial Circulation with Herbs

Susan Lin, my Chinese herbalist friend in New York, has developed a beauty mask using precious herbs such as myrrh, frankincense, and tang kuei. This facial pack increases surface circulation to renew skin freshness. You mix the powdered herbs with honey and egg white, apply the mask to your face, and let it dry. This is not a harsh skin peel, but feels like a delightful facial massage. Order the powder directly from Susan at Lin Sisters Herb Shop in New York (see the Herbal Access section at the back of the book).

You can make your own facial packs with a kitchen blender, combining foods that resurface and soothe the skin. For example, blend cucumber, papaya, and potato into a puree. Strain the puree and set the liquid aside. Apply the mashed ingredients to your face. Lie down for fifteen minutes and feel the cooling tingle from the enzymes and potassium in the mixture. You can also add raw oatmeal and scrub your face with the mashed ingredients. Rinse off with warm water and splash on what's left of the liquid cucumber, papaya, and potato.

## A Pleasure Cure

A leisurely soak in a warm tub will not only relax your muscles but will change your outlook when you add healing herbs.

### Spa bath

For the evening, transform your bath into your healing space. Take an hour. Light candles and incense and turn out the lights. Play a tape of ocean or woodsy sounds as you fill the tub with hot water and Epsom salts. Put a mineral clay mask on your face and spread it down the center of your chest to the solar plexus, the area beneath your heart where the ribs end and the stomach begins.

As you soak, rub Epsom salts into the soles of your feet. Drink a warm tea made from steeping two bay leaves and a slice of raw ginger in a cup of water.

When you have relaxed completely, imagine you are in a forest pond. Are you a fish? Gently inhale and puff up. Then exhale, letting your tension leave like the quiver of a fish's tail through your feet. Are you a frog? Lying flat, slowly fill your abdomen as you inhale, while drawing up your knees. Then as you exhale, straighten your legs in the water.

Fishes and frogs have desires too. What do you wish to do as a frog or fish that you have never done before? Something simple, easy to attain in your warm pond. Give yourself time to see it, feel it, and have it.

Nature's medicines will work to create health and beauty whether or not you believe in them. Miracles can happen by freeing trapped vitality to follow its destined course. The foods in this chapter make you younger because they help healing proceed smoothly. They reduce stress and ennui and wash away old unproductive patterns.

Total youth is more than bright eyes and dewy skin. It is a fresh outlook gained from being open to pleasure. The culmination of your wisdom, kindness, and strength shows through your relaxed smile.

## Five healing baths for glowing skin

These baths do more than make bubbles: they stimulate energy to create a fresh, lovely complexion. Use only a few drops of the recommended essential oils because they have a powerfully stimulating effect. Take the five different baths following this order on five consecutive evenings. Soak for twenty minutes, while sipping a warm, healing brew such as green tea to which you have added mint leaves and crushed coriander seeds.

To a tub of hot water add one of the following:

1. 20 ounces baking soda and ½ cup iodized salt
2. 16 ounces of hydrogen peroxide and pure essential clove oil

3. 2 quarts apple cider vinegar and pure essential rosemary oil
4. 16 ounces witch hazel and pure essential jasmine oil
5. 1 cup Epsom salts and pure essential rose oil

---

# A Ten-Day Program for Clear, Glowing Skin

Follow this program daily and make new skin in ten days.

## Daily Skin Supplements

Vitamins A, E, beta carotene including Omega 3 fish oils taken at the same time as evening primrose or borage oil

A balanced combination of B complex vitamins

At least 2,000 mg vitamin C, along with flavonoids and rutin

100 mg zinc with mixed minerals, including copper and gold

Alternate five doses each homeopathic ferrum phos. 6x strength and kali. sulph. 6x along with sulphur 6x to oxygenate the skin

If constipated add homeopathic nat. sulph. 6x to the above homeopathic remedies or a laxative such as cascara sagrada or malva tea at bedtime

## Daily Herbs

½ cup aloe vera gel added to apple juice or green tea, along with 1 capsule myrrh and ¼ teaspoon turmeric powder

A tea made from simmering 1 handful each of dandelion herb and honeysuckle flowers for 15 minutes. Drink 2 or more cups of this laxative brew unsweetened. Regulate the dosage as needed.

Or simmer 1 handful honeysuckle flowers, and with each cup take 4 capsules dandelion to clear eczema and acne in about one week

6 capsules gotu kola and 3 of sarsaparilla between meals

## Foods

Avoid hot spices and fried foods.

Drink a glass of Pineapple Protein Drink for breakfast.

Fix a bowl of barley soup, adding parsley, mint, tarragon, or cumin.

Eat at least one salad and lots of green and yellow vegetables.

Have almond milk or Spinach Zest Drink before bed (see pages 57 and 60).

## *Daily Skin Brushing*

See page 140 for the benefits of skin brushing. Always avoid the face and use a soft natural-fiber brush or loofah intended only for the skin. Brush in large strokes downward from head to foot. Reduce chronic facial redness by brushing down the solar plexis (the area between the breasts) to the stomach, legs, and insteps. Foot massage also calls the body's circulation downward, removing inflammation from the face.

---

# Keys

Acne and eczema: zinc, dandelion-honeysuckle tea, Lien Chiao Pai Tu Pien or homeopathic kali. mur., kali. sulph., calc. sulph., and silicea

Warts: homeopathic thuja occidentalis.

Graying and falling hair: Fo-ti (he shou wu), han lian cao

Wrinkles: astragalus and jujube date tea and elixir.

Bags and circles under the eyes: see candida, page 155

# Links: Chapters 3, 8 (spring and autumn), 11, 12, 13

# CHAPTER 6

# Computer-Related Stress and Pain

*Pain is frozen energy: warm it and be free.*

---

*Your Goal:* To unlearn painful work habits. To cure computer-related pain and poor circulation at home, at work, and in a traffic jam.

*Materials:* Rub-on pain relief—Tiger Balm, White Flower analgesic oil, Boswellin Cream; cooling foods and herbs that reduce congestion and water retention—asparagus, white potato, carrots, parsley, red cabbage, celery and celery seeds, chicory coffee substitute, aloe vera gel, and myrrh; homeopathic remedies that eliminate joint, tendon, and muscle pains—choose from homeopathic ferrum phos., calc. fluor., ruta grav., rhus. tox, arnica montana, and nat. phos.

---

It's midsummer 1998 as I write this. Radio and television promotion of *Asian Health Secrets* is still going strong. I'm exhausted but happily living in Vermont for the summer, trying renewal recipes that make me look and feel better than I have all year. I've started to lose the extra weight I put on while writing. (See Chapter 9.) My most pressing renewal issues now are the stubborn side effects of using my computer: the stiff neck, painful legs, carpal tunnel syndrome, and dim vision that come from sitting for hours staring at a screen. Pain is trapped circulation. Move your energy and blood circulation, and the healing process can begin.

Over the years, we have made great progress in healing physical and emotional pain. Our ancestors used powerful opiate drugs such as laudanum and liquor to stupefy their aches. Emotional laundry was washed clean at church or on the psychoanalyst's couch. Eventually, therapists realized that to cure pain, it had to be moved away from where it was trapped. From the 1960s through the 1980s, act-out therapies were in vogue. We had group screaming, rebirthing, est, then the recovery groups and twelve-steppers. Alcoholics Anonymous and its offshoots are still around. Why hasn't someone started SWA: Screen Watchers Anonymous? We need creative deprogramming—ways to unlearn painful computer habits.

Stress injuries are hard to fix because they are repetitive. Bad posture and improper clothes or movements can harm athletes as well as computer jockeys. Poor habits are easy to come by: I wrote my first book sitting on a piano stool. When I'm away from home, my trusty laptop and I find whatever setup we can work with. I doubt that I'll ever find the perfect angle for my arms, wrists, and eyes to approach the screen. One solution is to take herbs internally and smear them on externally to relieve tension and fatigue.

Another complication of computer injury is that since it is often nerve-related, we feel it more when we're under psychological stress. In your work situation, for example, do you have a boss or co-worker who is driving you nuts? Do you feel various aches worse just from being near that person? You may not be able to leave the job or a traffic jam, but I can recommend things you can do anywhere to ease tension and pain.

# Painful Stiff Neck, Shoulders, and Back

Any area of the body with impaired circulation is likely to have chronic muscle and joint pain. Arthritis can be another complication resulting from poor diet and weakness. Moving stuck circulation to bring more blood and oxygen to painful areas often temporarily relieves stress. The brain no longer reads "spasm" but instead reads "movement." Massage therapists, acupuncturists, and chiropractors can do a lot to help relieve pain. One basic principle involved in getting stuck energy to move is to vary the kind of stimulation. You might apply hot and cold packs to painful areas to move circulation, but there are easier ways.

## Oils and Plasters as Rub-On Cures

White Tiger Balm, Red Tiger Balm, and White Flower analgesic oil are Asian household pain remedies for quick, easy relief of pain and stiffness. Apply them to sore or stiff areas, as shown below, avoiding eyes and other delicate tissues. The evergreen ingredients in these salves and oils, which include menthol, wintergreen, and camphor, clear your senses with a refreshing spicy aroma and, depending on the variety you choose, will feel hot or will flash hot and then cold.

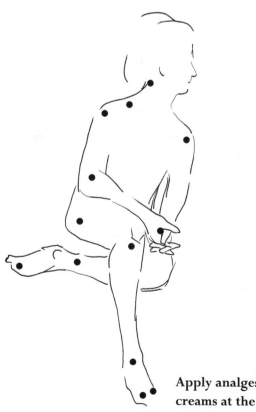

**Apply analgesic oils and creams at the points shown.**

Red Tiger Balm contains hot spices such as cinnamon and cajuput, which take the heating action deep into muscles and joints. This is fine for dull headaches, spasms, or neuralgia pains increased by cold weather. You know you need it if a heating pad sounds like a good idea.

Boswellin Cream, made by Nature's Herbs, is a hot, penetrating cream with a mild spicy fragrance. The heating ingredients in this health food store arthritis remedy are methyl salicylate and capsaicin along with Boswellia serrata, an East Indian form of turmeric that increases circulation.

White Tiger Balm and White Flower oil are another matter. Spreading these white analgesics onto stiff joints at shoulders, arms, or legs will flash hot and cold waves that increase circulation, a bit like taking a sauna followed by a dip in an ice-cold lake. They are made in Hong Kong and are available in Asian shops, food markets, and many health food stores. My drawing, based on Chinese acupuncture meridians, shows you the best places to apply analgesic balms and oils. Dab a drop of these hot-cold ointments also at the lower back and behind the knees.

# Help for Tired Legs

You may not actually have enlarged and discolored varicose veins, but only tired, swollen legs from stashing them under a desk. Other discomforts may include constipation, cracks on soles of your feet, or hemorrhoids. All these can be eliminated with a diet of fresh vegetables, fruits, grains, raw seeds, and warm green tea, adding lots of aloe vera gel or juice—up to one-half cup daily. If problems persist try the following remedies.

## Varicose Veins

Varicose veins can be improved by eliminating water retention in the legs, while enhancing local circulation with laxative and diuretic foods and stimulant herbs. Try this unusual but quite effective combination.

### Asparagus Legs Juice

Did you ever want your legs to be like fresh, firm, crisp asparagus? This raw juice, high in valuable plant calcium, magnesium, potassium, vitamins A, C, B-complex, iron, and necessary trace minerals, will do the trick. It provides rutin, a major bioflavonoid, to keep the capillaries flexible. Juice the ingredients fresh each time.

**1 part raw asparagus**
**1 part white potato, with skin**
**1 part carrots, adding some of the green tops**
**1 part celery**
**1 handful fresh parsley**

No matter what your job is, if you've spent long hours sitting, leg circulation will be a chronic problem. Lack of exercise also weakens digestion, so be conservative with this powerful raw juice. Start with only ⅛ cup of the mixture. Then very gradually work up to no more than one 8-ounce glass daily, using the same proportions. Too much raw potato too fast can give you a splitting headache. Drink the juice fresh after lunch or dinner for two weeks or until you notice improvement. This juice cleanses the body and blood by stepping up elimination.

If juicing is too much trouble, try this simple recipe for good results. Add ½ cup aloe vera gel to water or apple juice and swallow it with 2 capsules myrrh twice daily. I recommend this combination throughout the book for various problems. It has broad beneficial effects because aloe is cooling and cleansing, while myrrh helps dissolve impurities. Aloe has been traditionally recommended for hemorrhoids, constipation, and inflamed internal or external tissue. Take the weight off your legs with these herbs that improve leg circulation. You can add aloe to green tea in order to strengthen and add elasticity to blood vessels at the same time.

Several companies make horse chestnut seed extract for varicose veins. It is not recommended for persons with liver or kidney problems or those who have had a stroke or heart disease, but for most people horse chestnut capsules can lower leg swelling by improving the circulation in leg veins. Reduce the dosage or discontinue use of any circulation stimulant if nausea, gastric irritation, or uncomfortable heartbeat occurs.

## Cracks in the Skin on Hands and Feet

For cracked skin on hands and feet, caused by poor circulation and weak internal organs, add one dose of homeopathic calc. fluor. 6x (calcium fluoride) to a cup of water and sip it five times daily. This form of calcium is a fortifier of weak, tired people—worthwhile because cow's milk calcium is so hard to absorb, and few of us eat enough green vegetables.

# Carpal Tunnel Syndrome

This most common computer injury can start as a slight twinge of pain or stiffness between the tendons on the inside of your wrist. For the unwise who ignore early warnings, it can become intense paralyzing agony. Jarring from repeated use of certain fingers or an awkward angle (where your wrist is lower than your fingers while computing) moves tension and stress injury up the arm. The result is carpal tunnel syndrome—an injured wrist, which can lead to tendonitis at the wrist and elbow, a stiff shoulder, and possibly even dislocated cervical vertebrae in your neck.

Mine started while I was writing *Asian Health Secrets* and did not heal until I had followed my carpal tunnel protocol for two weeks. The diet that works best for me is a combination of selected raw vegetable juices, herbs, and homeopathic remedies for tendonitis, arthritis, and fatigue.

If you follow my directions, you should be able to get rid of your carpal tunnel inflammation, or at least greatly reduce it, within one month. Considering the high cost and inconvenience of the somewhat risky surgical procedure often recommended for this malady, the natural way is well worth your time and trouble. Besides, part of my anti–carpal tunnel diet resembles others I recommend for cancer, heart trouble, and cellulite.

Like most people suffering from carpal tunnel syndrome, I hoped the condition would go away. It did after a month in the sun and hot mineral waters of California last winter, but soon it came back with the usual pain and numbness of the right hand. Early on, my discomfort was worse from 5:30 A.M. to about 7:00 A.M. Eventually it appeared any time I was fatigued.

According to traditional Chinese doctors, who centuries ago observed the functioning of acupuncture meridians, the two hours surrounding dawn are the time of day when adrenal energy is the lowest, when you are most prone to adrenal fatigue. Because adrenal vitality and heart function are interrelated, this is a time when many weak people die of heart failure. This information allowed me to begin to solve the problem of my carpal tunnel syndrome like a detective.

## Carpal Tunnel and Fatigue

If the wrist and arm pain and numbness are worse at dawn, after you've been out in the cold or eaten lots of cold raw food, or after diarrhea, the syndrome is a function of adrenal exhaustion. Also you may have become so weak that your posture has slumped enough to put extra stress on your vertebrae and spinal fluid. This often happens after you have worked for hours on your computer or you've been stuck in long traffic jams. The best remedies for this form of carpal tunnel syndrome are herbal tonics for fatigue and poor circulation. Some herbs can increase and coordinate both adrenal and heart energy for exhaustion. Others can help digestive energy when necessary. The following protocol offers suggestions that will work for anyone's carpal tunnel pain affecting wrist, arm, or neck. If they do not quiet your nerve pain after one week, you probably have a pinched nerve and should consult a chiropractor. My diet and herb recommendations for carpal tunnel syndrome are followed by additional help for people who work under constant negative stress, which can affect nerves and vision.

Post copies of the Carpal Tunnel Protocol and the I Hurt! box on page 89 at home, at work, and in your car. You can take the herbs and homeopathic remedies and smear on the herbal painkillers anywhere—even in the middle of Los Angeles traffic. See the drawing on page 83 to find sensitive massage areas. Turn a traffic jam into a healing experience.

---

## Carpal Tunnel Protocol

*After meals and at 10:00 A.M.:* 1 capsule hawthorn to strengthen the heart muscle and reduce poor circulation and fatigue.

*Between Meals:* **For improved mobility and less pain, add one dose (or 10 pills) of homeopathic ruta. grav. 30c strength to 1 quart water. This homeopathic form of garden rue reduces tendonitis. Drink it throughout the day, waiting twenty minutes after meals or coffee.**

Take to work a thermos of Red-Hot Juice (see page 85) to reduce pain, stiffness, and swelling. Drink one or two glasses along with digestive herbs at lunch or during the afternoon.

Take three or more doses of one of the following combinations:
ArthPlus, made by Nature's Herbs
Mobility 3, made by Health Concerns in Oakland
Ar-Ease Caps, made by Crystal Star, or any similar herbal combination designed to ease pain, reduce acid, and increase circulation

*Medicated Oils:* **Smear one drop of Tiger Balm White Flower oil or Boswellin Cream on the areas marked in the hand and arm drawing for carpal tunnel syndrome, found on page 83.**

---

# Carpal Tunnel: Additional Special Problems

## *Adrenal weakness and low enthusiasm*

You will need an energy tonic if joint and muscle pain is made worse by poor sleep, overwork, or cold weather. Increasing circulation with the herbs and homeopathic potions I recommend will help somewhat, but faced with adrenal fatigue and weakness, you will still suffer from lower backache, poor enthusiasm, frequent urination, diarrhea, or depression. One of my favorite energy tonics does more than stimulate energy. It actually builds strength and endurance by protecting your adrenal glands, those painful spots just above the kidneys. It is called Sexoton. You will read about it in Chapter 13, Total Energy for Work and Play.

## *Nervous upset or anxiety*

If your carpal tunnel symptoms seem worse after coffee, stress, aggravation, or cold drafts, they are likely related to nerve irritation and should be treated with a nervine, an herbal painkiller for raw nerves. Among the best

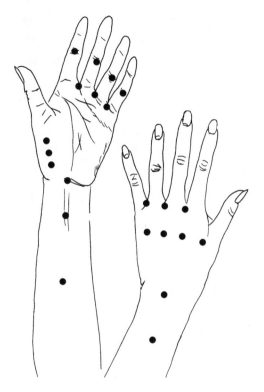

**Massage these spots for carpal tunnel syndrome.**

are a homeopathic combination called Neuritis #122 made by Borneman. It contains homeopathic magnesium, potassium, Bryonia alba, Rhus toxicodendron (rhustox.), and hypericum, and is recommended for tingling, burning pain, and numbness aggravated by cold, dampness, or overexertion.

If you drink coffee, a favorite hyperacidic nerve stimulant, a good way to come down from the ceiling and fall asleep is to take homeopathic coffee at bedtime. Homeopathic coffee cruda 30c rids your body of java's jump. You might add either of these homeopathic remedies to a cup of warm water or non-caffeine tea.

Another great way to quiet your nerves, reduce carpal tunnel pain, and ensure better sleep is, on an empty stomach, to take one or two capsules of evening primrose oil along with your daily dose of healthy Omega 3 fish oils. I like cod liver oil capsules. That combination ensures that the anti-inflammatory primrose is in your body at the same time as the fish oils, which soothes your overworked liver. Try it before bed and you may be surprised to experience tranquil, pleasant dreams.

# Pain Prevention Teas for Home and the Office

To avoid feeling as though you have been beaten up from work, take some preventive measures at home and at the office. First, avoid excess acid, which weakens joints and jangles the nerves. The caffeine in coffee, black tea, and chocolate increases arthritis pain and stiffness. Drinking coffee removes important nutrients, including calcium, from the body with every cup. This sets you up for arthritis even if you don't own a computer. A tasty coffee substitute is roasted chicory root.

### Chicory Espresso

Boil a strong mixture for one minute, using one tablespoon of roasted chicory per cup water. Drain it through a sieve, and the liquid will taste a bit like espresso. Then, if you like bitter espresso, add a pinch of turmeric powder, which increases circulation. Another good addition to a coffee substitute is powdered cardamom, a semisweet seed that stimulates energy and digestion. Add one pinch to each cup of hot chicory drink.

The best herbal sweetner to reduce joint aches and nerve-related pain is a Chinese remedy, Essence of Tienchi Flower Instant Beverage. See page 70.

# Herbal and Homeopathic Pain and Stiffness Preventers

Certain herbs and homeopathic remedies should be kept in your car and work space to prevent damage from poor circulation. Here are some drinks you can easily make to help ease pain and stiffness. The herbal brews are best used between meals. Wait twenty minutes after eating or drinking coffee before using homeopathic remedies.

For stiff shoulders, add one-quarter teaspoon each of cinnamon and turmeric powder per cup hot water. Drink it hot. Wrap the area with a scarf to protect your neck and shoulders from air conditioning.

For old injuries or arthritic stiffness anywhere in the body, add one dose of homeopathic rhus tox. 30c strength to a quart of spring water and sip it throughout the day. This homeopathic strength of poison ivy has a very different effect from the plant. It increases circulation, warming the joints. Rhus tox. 30c works best for stress or arthritis pains that feel better with movement and application of heat.

For dull aches and pains from severe exhaustion, add one dose of homeopathic arnica montana 30c strength per cup hot water and sip it occasionally for a few hours. Homeopathic arnica, a daisy, is normally used to heal bruises, but it is also recommended when you feel as though you've been beaten up.

# Supercleansing

People who spend hours sitting need special help ridding the body of congestion, fat, and unhealthy deposits in the muscles and at the joints. They need to supercleanse. Here's a tangy raw vegetable juice I've used this summer to get my joints and waistline back into shape. It helps arthritis, obesity, constipation, poor circulation, and painful puffy legs.

## Letha's Red-Hot Juice

¼ red cabbage
4 large celery stalks with leaves
¼ teaspoon celery seed
2 large carrots
¼ medium-size white onion (optional)
⅛ teaspoon prepared horseradish (optional)
½-inch slice raw ginger

**1 big handful fresh parsley**
**1 big handful fresh mint or 1 teaspoon dried**
**Juice of ½ lemon**

Juice all the ingredients together. It's best sipped during the afternoon. You might take a thermos to work. As with all raw juices, I recommend that you start by drinking only a small amount that you can easily tolerate. Or make a meal of it by adding popped corn and goat cheese.

This drink is spicy and very cleansing. People with red burning joints or other signs of inflammatory arthritis should use only red cabbage, celery, and celery seeds. Red cabbage, onion, and all parts of celery are wonderful for reducing joint pain from arthritis, but their pungent flavor makes it hard to drink them alone. Parsley reduces water retention, while ginger and horseradish eliminate chronic catarrh congestion.

It's a bad idea to drink raw juice first thing in the morning because the cold raw vegetables are difficult to digest. Instead, start the day with a cup of hot green tea, adding digestive herbs and spices such as ginger and mint.

# Painful Eyes and Poor Vision

After you have stared into a screen for years, you may see why it's called a terminal. Herbs can help massage your eyes from the inside, easing puffiness and eyestrain. Cloudy vision will improve when you start to take herbs internally that bring needed moisture to your eyes. That is the wonder of traditional Asian medical herbal combinations: they take the healing power of the herbs where they are most needed.

## Flowers for Your Eyes

For tired, bloodshot eyes, lumps under the jaw or in the neck, or hyperactivity with brain chatter from stress, fatigue, and poor circulation, brew a tea with prunella *(Prunella vulgaris),* a common weed. You can grow your own or order it dried from Chinese herbal merchants. In Chinese it's called xia ku cao. Add a handful of dried herb to a quart of water, simmer it for ten minutes, and refrigerate it for up to three days. It tastes blah. It's supposed to taste blah. If you spice it up with sugar or honey, it spoils the effects. If you find it dreadfully dull, add mint. If you have hypertension, add Essence of Tienchi Flowers Instant Beverage.

For cloudy vision, dry eyes, pounding headaches, or congestion from dust and pollen, brew a delicious sweet tea from Chinese chrysanthemum flowers. They are dried, small, round, yellowish flowers often seen in Chinese groceries and herb shops. They taste wonderful. No need for sweetener. They lift your spirits and clear simple cloudy vision after a cup or two taken between meals. You can order some from the Chinese herbal merchants listed at the back of this book.

## Vision-Strengthening Tea

Finally, here's a beneficial combination of herbs that refresh and moisturize eyes while protecting vision. It combines an energy herb with a blood tonic herb useful for eyestrain and weak vision. You might alternate this drink with chrysanthemum flower tea.

This is not technically a tea but an herbal decoction because you have to simmer the ingredients in water for twenty minutes instead of steeping them. Use one handful each of false ginseng (dang shen) and fructus lychii (also called lycium fruit, matrimony fruit, or gou ji tse).

Found in Chinese groceries and herb shops, dang shen resembles dried twigs, and lycium fruits are dried, small red berries that are sweet and sour, delicious enough to eat by themselves. If you eat a handful or two or add them to hot tea, you will feel as though pressure is leaving your eyes while they become more moist. The berries have a laxative effect if you eat too many.

Dang shen lifts your energy to treat prolapse problems. By cooking lycium fruit along with dang shen, you ensure that the moistening, blood-building effects of the fruit are taken to where they are most needed—

the eyes. If demands on your vision are constant, these herbs can help prevent fatigue and poor vision.

Any of these herbs, homeopathic remedies, and oils will improve
computer-related discomfort, but you'll get the best results by combining them in order to treat a number of related problems, as I have
done in the carpal tunnel protocol on page 81. You will reduce pain
while protecting yourself from further injury. Then you and your computer can ride off into the sunset, free and happy to face each other
another day.

---

## ⚮   Ten-Day Program to Ease   ⚮
## Computer-Related Pain

*Day One to Day Six:* **At 10:00 A.M. take one capsule hawthorn
to increase circulation. Follow lunch and dinner with one capsule
hawthorn.**

Add 1 cup aloe vera gel to 1 quart spring water along with 10
pills each of homeopathic iron (ferrum phos. 6x), homeopathic
sodium phosphate (nat. phos. 6x), and homeopathic ruta grav. 6x.
Sip this mixture throughout the day between meals. The aloe, iron,
and ruta are anti-inflammatory, and homeopathic nat. phos. helps
remove uric acid from the joints.

Drink one glass of Red-Hot Juice daily. Start slowly!

Rub White Flower medicated oil or any such oil that flashes hot
and cold sensations into painful, stiff areas such as joints, neck, and
shoulders.

*Day Seven:* **Use only 10 pills homeopathic rhus. tox. 6x added to
1 quart spring water. Sip it between meals to warm joints and
increase circulation.**

Twice daily rub either red or white Tiger Balm or Boswellin
Cream into stiff areas, including neck, shoulders, and knees.

If you can tolerate the heat, take a home sauna by wrapping
up painful joints with kitchen plastic wrap and terry-cloth towels

to induce strong sweating. Then drink a cup or two of cinnamon tea.

*Day Eight and Day Nine:* **Repeat what you did on days one through six.**

*Day Ten:* **Repeat what you did on day seven.**

---

# I Hurt!

Hot burning pain; throbbing headaches; fever: homeopathic belladonna 30c

Heavy, dull aches; stuffed sinuses; sinus headaches; stomach distention; and pain that feels better with massage: homeopathic pulsatilla 30c

Stiffness or arthritis; pain that feels better with warmth and movement: homeopathic rhus. tox. 30c

Bruises; entire body feels as though you've been beaten: homeopathic arnica montana 30c

Tendons feel stretched, aching or burning: homeopathic ruta grav. 30c or 6x

Lower back and legs ache; poor circulation; cracks on hands or feet; weakness: homeopathic calc. fluoride 30c or 6x

Gout; severe burning and shifting pain in fingers or feet: homeopathic formica ruf 6x

*Your Medicine Cabinet:* **These homeopathic remedies are easy to find in health food stores and better supermarkets. Tear out this page to post as a guide. Homeopathic remedies are used at different strengths and dosages, according to the severity of the problem.**
    30c for acute problems
    6x for chronic problems, although for acute problems it can be taken every fifteen minutes.

---

# Keys

Spasm: aloe vera gel in green tea or apple juice

Eyestrain: Prunella vulg. tea plain or added to green tea

Varicose veins: aloe vera gel, horse chestnut capsules

Indigestion: ginger, mint, tarragon, and green tea

Nervousness and low energy: gotu kola capsules, homeopathic kali. phos. 30c or gelsemium 30c

Tendonitis: homeopathic ruta grav. 30c (see carpal tunnel syndrome, page 80)

**Links:** Also see Chapters 8, 11, 13

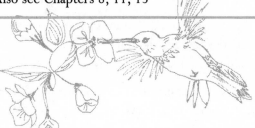

# CHAPTER 7

# Brilliant Comebacks

*Illness and injury are*
*opportunities for renewal.*

---

*Your Goal:* **Regain vitality after serious injury or illness.**
*Materials:* **Anti-stress vitamins and minerals; herbs and homeopathic remedies that calm the mind such as gotu kola, Siberian ginseng, and homeopathic aconite; pain and wound remedies, including homeopathic ledum, hypericum, and Chinese Yunnan Paiyao; anti-candida herbs—Australian tea tree oil taken with homeopathic belladonna; homeopathic carbo veg. for indigestion; Chinese Xiao Yao Wan or Curing Pills for nausea; eclipta alba for hair loss after chemotherapy and astragalus to rebuild resistance and counter fatigue. A cheerful, positive attitude also works wonders.**

---

Illness and injury are weakening and aging. If you know how to bounce back after acute discomforts, your vitality will not be compromised. Change your attitude toward the discomfort and you can use your recovery time to great advantage. Have you recently had an accident or surgery? Have you experienced depression after childbirth? Have your looks been damaged by substance addictions or a chemotherapy cocktail? You need to bounce back as quickly as possible. This chapter will help you make a brilliant comeback after the shocks and healing pains of fate and modern life. You can order the following healing nostrums from the companies listed in the Herbal Access section of this book.

# Step One: Be Prepared

You can't always predict injury, but you can be certain to recover quickly if you prepare. The following protocol works well for dental work, surgery, or simple puncture wounds. It pays to strengthen vitality and enhance circulation beforehand and take steps to clear swelling, bruising, inflammation, and pain afterward.

For at least one month prior to periodontal dental work or surgery, stop smoking and drinking alcohol as much as possible. Taking 3,000 to 6,000 mg time-release vitamin C with bioflavonoids daily will strengthen blood vessels, help prevent infection, and reduce inflammation. But you should stop taking large doses of vitamin C one week prior to surgery. Extra vitamin C then thins the blood and may encourage bleeding. If you usually experience excess bleeding, take 60 mg vitamin K, a natural coagulant, daily for one week prior to surgery. During the weeks prior to surgery, drink extra water and take vitamins; minerals, including 100 mg zinc; and trace minerals, including copper.

If possible, get a good massage once or twice a week to improve circulation. That will speed healing because your body will be ready to eliminate surgery drugs and heal bruises faster.

Try to get extra sleep and take a natural tonic especially for your nerves. Here are a few suggestions. Take at least six gotu kola capsules daily between meals. Gotu kola heals nerve tissue and the brain itself for better concentration and memory while it calms you. A low-dose form of Siberian ginseng such as the Chinese-made liquid remedy Wuchaseng, is helpful. Take a teaspoon as needed daily and before bed. If you are nervous, insomniac, pale, and languid from anemia, take Calms Forte, a homeopathic remedy available in health food stores, containing iron and other helpful minerals to quiet anxiety. All these work well for chronic weakness and nervousness.

But if you panic at the thought of surgery—screaming, crying, restlessly pacing the floor, or shutting yourself in at home—homeopathic aconite 30c (monkshood) will settle your nerves. It is used for sudden high fever, shock, fright, hysteria, and anxiety attacks. If you become overly sensitive to light, noise, and touch; if crowds or darkness alarms you, or if you are filled with a sense of impending doom or evil, homeopathic aconite 30c is required. Take one dose every half hour until you feel calm and begin to perspire; then stop taking the remedy. Repeat only as needed every four hours. Homeopathic aconite 30c will not cloud your thinking or memory the way a sedative drug might. Homeopathic aconite is also recommended for early stages of colds when the onset is sudden and the symptoms make you fearful.

# Step Two: Speed Healing

Natural pain and puncture wound remedies will help you recover your strength and morale quickly because they increase circulation and boost your natural defenses. Here are some ways you can use them before and after trauma.

## Nerve Pains

My dentists and their staff in Vermont are great. Unlike some people, the woman cleaning my teeth does not aspire to sing on Broadway: she actually gets excited about my teeth. You may not be so lucky. Dental treatments can give you an ouch for hours afterward. If your face hurts from cold or hot foods or weather, facial nerves have been irritated. You may feel that you want to wrap up your head and hide away under a blanket. There are better ways to treat nerve inflammation (neuritis).

Anti-inflammatory homeopathic combinations work very well because you can adjust the dosage to suit your needs. If the pain is intense, you can take a dose every fifteen minutes until it lets up. Then continue as needed with one dose every two hours or so. Sensitivity to heat also signals infection. Check with your dentist.

Neuritis is also the name of a remedy made from a combination of homeopathic apis ven. pur. 6x (bee venom) and magnesium phosphate 6x, made by Washington Homeopathic Products in Bethesda, Maryland. The homeopathic venom works the opposite way the bee sting would—it takes away swelling and pain. The remedy is recommended for nerve inflammation symptoms such as soreness, numbness or stiffness of nerves and muscles.

# Bleeding Gums and Puncture Wounds

After dental surgery or gum treatments have left you bleeding, bruised, and swollen, you need strong help. Homeopathic apis is indicated for puncture wounds that feel hot with stinging pains that feel better after applying ice. Homeopathic ledum (marsh tea) is used for puncture wounds with redness, swelling, and throbbing pain and when the wound feels cold to the touch but is relieved by cold or ice. Homeopathic hypericum (Saint John's wort) is useful for wounds that have sharp shooting pains. Besides lessening pain, especially in areas richly supplied with nerves—fingers, toes, and spine—hypericum speeds up the healing process when used internally and externally.

Yunnan Paiyao (Yunnan white powder) is the Chinese herbal drug of choice for curing wounds, pain, and swelling after trauma. Spread directly on wounds and taken orally, it works like a combination of the above homeopathic remedies, which reduce inflammatory and noninflammatory swelling and pain. Like homeopathic arnica 30c, it also heals bruises. In addition, it stops hemorrhage. Throughout Asia it is used for deep injuries, including gunshot wounds. The capsules and powder are considered standard equipment for soldiers in the Chinese People's Army. Yunnan Paiyao also helps bring oozing skin infections to the surface to facilitate healing. I recommend taking Yunnan Paiyao just before dental treatments and surgery anywhere in the body.

The formula contains raw and steamed tienchi ginseng and other herbs that increase circulation to heal broken blood vessels. It quickly stops hemorrhage, internal bleeding, and pain. It even speeds the healing of broken bones. Yunnan Paiyao can save your life. Every emergency room and ambulance should carry this highly effective anti-hemorrhage remedy.

The powder comes in a small bottle or on a sheet containing a dozen capsules. Each package contains a tiny red ball used to treat severe injuries and bleeding such as gunshot wounds. Swallow the small red ball just prior to surgery: it will not interfere with surgery drugs.

After you awaken from surgery, take the capsules internally, according to directions, usually six to eight daily, two after each meal, until pain, bruising, and swelling subside. Continue it for two weeks, during which time you should eat a variety of warm, nourishing cooked foods, avoiding fish.

I have seen miraculous results with Yunnan Paiyao, including fast recovery from surgery, muggings, and car accidents. When I've recommended it for liposuction patients, their plastic surgeons have called me to rave about how well their patients healed. There is no reason why people have to hemorrhage to death with herbal medicines like this available! You can buy Yunnan Paiyao capsules in any Chinese grocery or herb shop. If you are not near a Chinatown, you can order it from sources listed at the back of this book.

# Step Three: Give Yourself Time to Heal

Use the time necessary to heal after surgery as a rejuvenating rest from work and worry. Make it a time of renewal. Tell everyone you are too tired to see them. If you really are too tired, try one of the natural energy boosters from Chapter 13. Also useful are Recovery Pills made by Seven Forests. Your health food store can order them from suppliers listed in the Herbal Access section. They contain Chinese tonic herbs, some of which build blood and increase energy—rehmannia, tang kuei, ginseng, peony, eucommia, epimedium, and clove—and others that strongly increase circulation for reducing pain and numbness—agkistrodon (a snake), cinnamon bark, cyperus, myrrh, and lindera. This could be used with Yunnan Paiyao for weak people who need to build themselves up after serious illness, surgery, childbirth, and shock. It helps arthralgia, stiff shoulders, and general weakness. It should not be used with fever because it's warming. If you are chilled and weak, you can take it regularly, three or four pills at a time with a little wine, to enhance blood circulation.

You can transform your downtime into a beauty cure. Taking Yunnan Paiyao, homeopathic arnica 6x, or Seven Forest's Recovery Pills will facilitate circulation throughout the body. That will help dissolve the effects of poor circulation—cellulite and fibroids. If you combine these wound-healing remedies with the appropriate cleansing and weight loss diet and massage from Part Three, you will go a long way toward getting your body and mind into shape. Do this regularly for prevention.

# Recovery from Modern Medicines

## Candida

If antibiotics, birth control pills, rich foods, and stress have given you candida, a yeast, use one drop of Australian Tea Tree Oil as toothpaste. Its antifungal-antiyeast action is effective for internal and external use. Add one drop of this bracing, refreshing oil to a cup of hot tea to clear your head of cobwebs. Some say it smells like floor wash. While the yeast is dying, you will crave all the things that make it grow, especially fruits, alcohol, and bread. You will likely get a headache as your body detoxifies. For sudden hot, throbbing withdrawal headaches use homeopathic belladonna 30c.

To eliminate all yeast symptoms, including low energy, poor concentration, spaciness, mood swings, and indigestion, you have to do more than use Australian Tea Tree Oil. For two or three days while using the antiyeast remedy, you have to eliminate yeast bread and pastries, sweets, fruits, and fermented foods like pickles, tamari, and vinegar. Tofu and all soy products should temporarily be eliminated. Soft drinks, alcohol, refined sugar, and party foods all make yeast grow. Obviously, kill the yeast after the holidays.

For three days eat nothing but vegetables, rice cakes, steamed fish, and bottled water to help kill the yeast. You've got to be tough or you'll get cranky or develop chronic indigestion after taking antibiotics. The yeast wants to live, and it will make you crave everything you shouldn't eat while you are killing it. Do not give up. I have never met anyone who was cured of candida with drugs such as nystatin. But occasional use of Australian Tea Tree Oil along with a temporary change in your diet can correct the problem.

At the same time, add healthy bacteria for your colon in the form of powdered turmeric or acidophilus. That will allow you to destroy the yeast without too much trouble. Barring a fever, take ¼ teaspoon powdered turmeric in a cup of water, tea, or yogurt three times daily. This not only helps rebuild a healthy colon; it also helps regulate blood sugar.

Acidophilus is the best source of healthy bacteria you can find. Most health food stores sell milk-free acidophilus for persons who are lactose-intolerant. Some people say the best way to absorb acidophilus is directly in the colon as a suppository once a day. If you take the capsules orally, use a total of four daily, one taken one half hour before meals and at bedtime.

If you still have indigestion and stomach gurgling, take a few doses of homeopathic carbo veg. 30c, a digestible form of charcoal that absorbs gas bubbles. Use it fifteen minutes after meals or as needed.

---

## A Five-Day Anti-Candida Plan

*Morning:* **If you drink coffee at breakfast, wait twenty minutes before using any homeopathic remedy. Take acidophilus one half hour before eating.**

*Breakfast:* **One piece of sourdough bread, toasted, or rice cakes, steamed vegetables, some fish, or a boiled egg.**

*To kill the yeast:* **Have one cup of hot tea or water, adding one drop of Australian Tea Tree Oil and one dose of homeopathic belladonna 30c for headache or homeopathic carbo veg. 30c for indigestion. If you need extra help with digestion or blood sugar balance (hypoglycemia) add Xiao Yao Wan pills (see page 99) and chromium. For nausea add a slice of raw ginger to tea or chew it.**

*Lunch:* **Large vegetable salad, pasta with sauce and fresh herbs, vegetable enchilada, or soup. Hot tea. Nuts or pumpkin seeds.**

*Midafternoon:* **One drop of Australian Tea Tree Oil in vegetable juice.**

*Dinner:* **Eat a normal dinner but avoid fruits, bread, sweets, and alcohol. Before bed, take a capsule of acidophilus or one half teaspoon of turmeric powder in a cup of yogurt or in a cup of warm green tea.**

---

# Recovering from Chemotherapy

One option few people think of when considering cancer chemotherapy is—just don't do it. Although anticancer drugs have become de rigueur, in many cases there is evidence that chemotherapy sometimes does little good and can do extensive harm. One case in point is the recent reluctance of certain physicians to treat prostatitis with cancer drugs because of the devastating side effects, including chronic urinary incontinence and impotence. I've heard Dr. Robert Atkins, the famous diet doctor, say that prostate cancer should never be operated on. He said the results of prostate surgery, radiation, and chemotherapy are far worse than the disease. Instead of standard procedures, Dr. Atkins's clinic uses a regime of herbs to destroy the cancer. Although everyone requires individual care, this information gives pause for thought.

Over the years I have met a number of people diagnosed with cancer who were actively pursuing nutrition and herbs as their main treatment. They were bright, alert, optimistic, and improving physically while also building physical and emotional strength and reinforcing immunity. The key to their success is self-determination. The cleansing and invigorating health suggestions found in this book can help anyone interested in pursuing that choice. Building health is quite different from nonintervention. Natural cures acknowledge the fact that current Western medicine does not have all the answers. We each have the opportunity and responsibility to heal ourselves, using the best means available to us.

In Asia, Western drugs are considered too expensive, a medicine of last resort, or totally unnecessary. In Japan, herbal patent remedies like those made in China are available with a doctor's prescription because, after years of Western scientific laboratory testing, Japanese doctors trust herbal medicines. In Chinese hospitals where I have worked, traditional herbal pills such as those that follow are used to combat serious or so-called incurable illnesses along with the fatigue, low immunity, and secondary illness associated with modern Western drugs.

## Nausea and Indigestion Resulting from Chemotherapy

Xiao Yao Wan, a Chinese patent remedy, offers digestive herbs such as ginger and mint along with blood- and immune-building herbs that soothe indigestion, settle the stomach, and fight depression. The digestive center is also our emotional center. When we're upset, we feel it in the solar plexus, abdomen, and heart. This combination of herbs in pill form is a convenient, fast-acting way to feel better in the stomach and chest because it normalizes digestion and local circulation. That in turn frees emotions from the tight knot we can feel just under the ribs. Use the small brown pills, from six to twelve per dose, at meals or anytime you feel pinched, suffocated, or hopelessly out of your center. They help to ease nausea and lack of appetite.

Bu Zhong Yi Qi Wan, another Chinese over-the-counter remedy, treats fatigue, chronic diarrhea, and low enthusiasm. It works well when chemotherapy has left you feeling empty and lifeless. Your tongue may look white- or gray-coated, indicating exhaustion and poor digestion. This remedy lifts your energy and strengthens your center. Take it with aloe if you are constipated. Otherwise, take a dose that feels right, anywhere from six to ten pills three or more times daily.

## Poor Immunity and Exhaustion after Chemotherapy

Astragalus has been touted as a major anticancer herb that builds immunity and vigor. Positive test results on it have been reported in the *Journal of the American Medical Association* and are available on the Internet as well as in the popular press. In China, certain forms of this pleasant semisweet herb are used to fight off cancer or retard its spread. The best way to use astragalus in conjunction with or after chemotherapy is to add one tablespoon of the powder to juice three times daily. You can also take the herb if you do not have cancer but wish to remain strong and free of colds and allergies in the fall and winter. (See pages 131–135 for more anticancer information.)

## Hair Loss after Chemotherapy

Some people I know have come to believe in Chinese herbs because they prevented or reversed hair loss resulting from cancer therapies. The commonly used formulas for this problem contain blood-building herbs because hair is considered to be an outcrop of healthy blood and bones.

Alopecia Areata Pills are Chinese combination pills containing Polygonum multiflori, rehmannia, Angelica sinensis, salvia, paeonia, schizandra, codonopsis, chaenomelis, and notopterygi. These herbs nourish blood, improve circulation, and improve hair growth. Use such moistening or blood-building formulas as soon after chemotherapy as possible, not during it.

Another single herb that regenerates bone marrow, thereby replenishing thinning hair, is han lian cao (Eclipta alba). This herb is useful, whether or not you have cancer, for hair loss from chemicals, illness, poor diet, or drug abuse. Have your favorite Chinese shop powder the herb for you. It tastes a bit like dried leaves, which it is, so you should fill empty capsules with the powder. Buy the capsules from a health food store and take six a day after meals. Within four to six weeks, you will notice new, strong, shiny hair. What's more, your liver, bone marrow, and blood will be reconditioned from han lian cao. If this cooling herb makes you feel chilled or weakened, take a dose of Xiao Yao Wan along with it.

## Weakness and Depression after Childbirth

One of life's greatest joys can lead to extreme depression resulting from exhaustion. This has little to do with your attitude toward motherhood.

It's normal to collapse while your body regroups from loss of strength and blood, but you can cut your recovery time to a fraction and reduce depression with herbs used by Chinese mothers. After you are home from the hospital or have taken herbs to clear the afterbirth, you can raise your energy and heal your internal wounds with Shih Chuan Da Bu Wan (Ten Inclusive Great Tonifying Pills), a Chinese patent remedy containing tang kuei, rehmannia, codonopsis, astragalus, atractylodes, paeonia root, poria fungus, licorice root, cinnamon bark, and ligusticum rhizome. The standard dosage is eight pills three times daily (24 pills or more as needed). These are energizing, blood-building tonic herbs that get you back on your toes. Take them for a month or more.

# Traveler's Corner: I Came, I Saw, I Caught It

Sometimes you have to make a brilliant comeback by killing germs or parasites, the result of unwise eating or foreign travel. For that purpose, there are many useful antibiotic, antiseptic, and cleansing herbs. When traveling, it's hard to avoid getting sick. Once I arrived in Ladakh to find a civil war in full swing, with tear gas, shootings, and martial law keeping people off the streets. In a situation like that you can be sure no one is worried about washing the dishes. You end up eating more than the chef prepared. On the other hand, you could be in a great restaurant somewhere with questionable water, forget yourself, and drink a glass of iced tea. No one boils water to make ice. The result, more often than not, is some sort of intestinal parasite. Most are caused by infested water or food prepared by dirty hands.

When you have parasites you feel lousy and develop weird eating habits. I remember the first time I got back from India, I couldn't look at the color green, listen to Indian music, or eat Indian food without feeling nauseated. My liver was overreacting from vindaloo stress caused by hot spices, and I had amoebas.

# Amoebas

Amoebas are one-celled parasites that hang out in the colon but can spread to the liver, lungs, and joints. They reproduce constantly so you can hardly get rid of them. They can cause excess mucus and severe diarrhea or jellylike stools, sometimes with cramps.

Rich, sweet, mucus-producing foods make them worse. After I got amoebas, I had to give up milk, red meat, alcohol, and creamy desserts. For months all I could eat were salads and baked potatoes. I lost fifteen pounds. It was a blessing in disguise. People started asking me how to catch the disease. I do not recommend it.

Parasites can make you very weak. Pretty soon you seem clogged with them. You feel that anyone who talks to you is somehow sucking your vitality. Or you imagine yourself oozing from place to place like a giant amoeba. It's creepy. With herbs I got over it.

For treating amoebas, Chinese goldenseal is the herb of choice among my Chinese friends. It comes as a powder or as tiny bitter pills. Take the pills according to the directions and use the powder to make a cleansing enema once daily. To make the enema, add one teaspoon of Chinese golden seal powder to one quart boiling water to make a tea. Strain it and let the water cool enough not to be irritating. I am lazy, though, and prefer using one tiny pill as a suppository when I have symptoms. That will keep the parasites in check as long as you change your diet, avoiding the mucus-producing foods that parasites enjoy.

---

# ❧ Fight Off Parasites by Maintaining ❧ a Healthy Colon

Avoid gooey sweets and dairy products

Eat antiparasite foods: radishes, carrots, garlic, and pumpkin seeds, along with an anticandida diet

Follow meals with one-half teaspoon turmeric powder added to water, tea, or rice milk, or use milk-free acidophilus

# Pill Remedies

Other antiparasite alternatives include both Eastern and Western drugs, several of which are banned in America but available over the counter in Asia and in Chinatowns everywhere. They work fast but can have side effects including candida (see page 96) or worse. Especially dangerous is Flagell, which reportedly can have damaging effects on the liver and kidneys, including cancer.

Herbal pills work well but slowly. They include several Chinese herbal combinations made by Seven Forests. Your health food store can order them for you from distributors such as Health Concerns. APP pharmacy in New York carries Seven Forest products.

Omphalia 11 works to destroy worms and giardia because it contains drying and antiseptic herbs, including omphalia, areca and torreya seed, mume, quisqualis, codonopsis, atractylodes, ginger, zanthoxylum, and raphanus. Licorice is added to help blend the other ingredients. Add other Seven Forests combinations such as Bupieurum S for abdominal bloating or Ginseng 18 for weakness with chronic diarrhea. Herb distributors do not give information on their products over the phone so you should consult a health expert at the same time.

In American health food stores you can find many antiparasite capsules that cleanse and recondition the colon. They often contain bitter and pungent herbs used to strip the colon of mucus such as black walnut hulls, garlic, gentian, butternut bark, prickly ash bark, wormwood, and cascara sagrada, a laxative.

Wormwood *(Artemisia apica)*, called ching hao in Chinese, is also used to lower fever in malaria. It's anti-inflammatory for the liver. Powdered wormwood can be combined with powdered clove and grapefruit seed, an astringent herb, to purge all sorts of parasites. To save money, have an Asian herb shop powder the herbs; then you can buy empty capsules from a health food store and fill them yourself.

For long-term prevention, I add antiparasite herbs to homemade digestive bitters. Use one to three ounces of herbal powder per quart of liquor, depending on the taste of the herbs. Steep the herbs in vodka for at least three weeks. The dosage is ten to twenty drops in a little water after meals. The alcohol will allow the herbs to work directly on your liver and digestive tract.

It's a basic belief in traditional Asian and American alternative medicine that cleansing the body of excess mucus and its by-products will help prevent congestive illnesses such as asthma, arthritis, allergies, cancer, and overweight. We don't necessarily get these conditions as we age, but they certainly age us.

With a little careful attention to your diet you can make a brilliant comeback in a few months. You won't be considered technically free of parasites until you test negative three consecutive times. If you take Western medical drugs recommended for parasites, you may never lose them but will very likely develop candida as a result. My diet and herb recommendations for those problems will make you feel better. Anti-mucus and anticandida herbs leave you feeling fresh, clean, and ready to travel again.

# Keys

Bruises, injury, and surgery: Yunnan Paiyao, homeopathic arnica montana 30c

Nerve pain and irritation: valerian tea or capsules

Yeast infections and thrush: Australian Tea Tree Oil along with homeopathic belladonna 30c

Chemotherapy nausea and weakness: Bu Zhong Yi Qi Wan, Curing Pills

Fright or shock after accident or injury: Rescue Remedy (homeopathic remedy)

Thirst and dehydration after fever: American ginseng tea

Links: Also see Chapters 13, 16

# CHAPTER 8

# Your Yearlong Rejuvenation Calendar

*There's a time for every herb under heaven.*

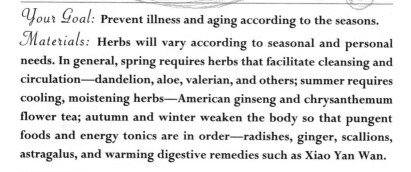

*Your Goal:* **Prevent illness and aging according to the seasons.**

*Materials:* **Herbs will vary according to seasonal and personal needs. In general, spring requires herbs that facilitate cleansing and circulation—dandelion, aloe, valerian, and others; summer requires cooling, moistening herbs—American ginseng and chrysanthemum flower tea; autumn and winter weaken the body so that pungent foods and energy tonics are in order—radishes, ginger, scallions, astragalus, and warming digestive remedies such as Xiao Yan Wan.**

M y approach to staying young and well is simple: I revitalize energy and beauty daily, and I prevent health problems before they occur. This eliminates worry and fear. I don't have to think about aging every minute. In fact, I enjoy prevention by using a special calendar.

This calendar begins in January, but you can begin your rejuvenation plan any month. A lot of people begin during the full moon or on their birthday. Each season of this calendar, like each section of the book, can stand alone to help you with specific problems such as overweight or low energy. I suggest that you follow my diet and herbal advice for the entire month, or at least for the first week of each month. Eventually you will want to add personalized remedies from other chapters. I begin each month of the calendar with a list of supplies you'll need. Substitutions are always possible, but try to maintain my herbal-energy recommendations—for example, don't use hot, spicy herbs when I recommend cooling bitter or sour ones.

You can lengthen or shorten the season according to your local weather. For that reason, at the beginning of each season I've described atmospheric conditions that apply and what you need to do about them. This will help you to understand the energy balance required for many different situations.

## Rejuvenation Plan for the Year

| Month | Goals | Herbal examples |
|---|---|---|
| January | Enhance sexuality | Ashwagandha, royal jelly |
| February | and vitality; | Ginger, clove, Sexoton |
| (Cold) | fortify | Oyster-shell calcium, |
|  |  | Pearl powder |
| March | Cleanse | Dandelion, aloe, myrrh |
| April | Weight loss | Tumor-dissolving herbs |
|  |  | Headache, arthritis herbs |
| May | Quiet nerves | Wuchaseng, gotu kola |
| (Humid) |  |  |
| June | Cool inflammation | American ginseng tea |
|  |  | Chrysanthemum flower tea |
| July | Cleanse impurities | Honeysuckle-dandelion tea |
| August | Weight loss | Tumor-dissolving herbs |
| (Hot) |  |  |
| September | Prevent colds and flu | Astragalus, radishes, |
| October |  | cinnamon, ginger, scallions |

| November | Build energy | Chinese ginseng, epimedium, and lycium |
| December (Cool, dry, or cold) | Prevent depression | Xiao Yao Wan, clove, cardamom |

The seasons create us. Spring is born of unquenchable desire. New life comes up green, fist first, and unfolds finger by finger. Young plants deep in pollen welcome bees buzzing from bud to bud, sweet perfume driving them wild. Summer flowers yield juicy fruits, saplings become strong trees. Blue-gray oceans churn the world. Wind-spun tides make the seasons. Not until autumn, with the silver moon set in sapphire, do we pause for reflection: "What has changed? What have I become?" Winter's sleep and dreams give rise to hope. It is a time to embrace our perfection and a time to woo lovers.

# How to Proceed

You might want to photocopy or post the current season's suggestions so that you can pay attention to the goals and supplies needed to ward off stress and fatigue related to the current weather conditions. Of course, the time and length of seasons will vary depending on where you live. Although I've composed this calendar according to New York's climate, roughly on the same latitude as Madrid, your weather will be similar at different times of the year.

It's most important that you know how to deal with atmospheric conditions that can harm the five elements. They are cold, wind, dampness, excess heat, and dryness. Cold weather weakens vitality. Wind irritates the nerves. Humidity slows digestion and elimination, which retards energy. Excess heat increases sweating, heart irregularities, and fever conditions. Dryness increases cough, thirst, dry skin, and anxiety.

# Winter

## January and February—The Pearl within the Oyster

*Weather:* Cold and raw with rain or snow

*Symptoms:* Extreme fatigue, weakness, low resistance, chills but without cold or flu symptoms, overwrought nervous anxiety

*Goals:* To build energy and vitality and to renew sexual strength

*Supplies:* Mixed trace minerals, oyster-shell calcium, pearl powder, raw sesame oil, Sexoton, Chinese ginseng, ginger, clove powder, cinnamon

*Herb of the Season:* Ashwagandha powder or capsules

*The Quick Fix:* Clove tea

*A Pleasure Cure:* Chyavanprash

*Special Problems:* Depression—Xiao Yao Wan, kava kava capsules; insomnia or palpitations—Homeopathic Calms Forte

Wintry weather requires herbs to sweat out chills, nutritional tonics that bolster energy and rejuvenate sexual vitality, and natural sedatives to calm the mind. Our capacity for love and vitality comes from a reservoir deep within us. The backbone of our compassion and courage comes from feeling secure, strong, and at ease. Minerals give us this assurance and grace because they protect bones, blood, and muscles, especially the heart muscle.

Calcium fortifies our framework of muscles and bones. Trace minerals make all the complicated functions of energy production possible. Warming digestive herbs and spices heal our emotional center by building a fire that processes foods and negative thoughts. Warming stimulant herbs for this season include adrenal tonics that rebuild our muscle strength while they gently increase metabolism.

## Plan for the Season

January and February are months when you will want to build up your reserves so that spring will explode with high energy. An early-to-bed schedule is in order. An afternoon nap is okay when necessary. Warm cooked foods with digestive and stimulant spices will add more sunshine to this dark part of the year.

## Winter teas

You may want to steep some of these spices to create hot teas. Choose one group at a time. With fresh herbs, you can use a larger quantity, but with dried herbs use only a pinch of each ingredient per cup of hot water. A good time to enjoy these stimulant teas is midmorning or midafternoon.

> Ginger, cardamom, and mint
>
> Sage
>
> One sprig rosemary
>
> Cinnamon, orange peel, and clove buds
>
> Green or oolong tea

If you prefer the taste of coffee, try brewing roasted chicory root as a substitute, then add the spices. Chicory is a bitter herb that clears the skin of blemishes and helps maintain a healthy liver. If you make it strong—one tablespoon chicory per cup of water, simmered for about one minute—it tastes like espresso.

## Winter foods

Warm cooked foods that are low in animal protein and fat include tofu, grains, seeds, nuts, and dried fruits; high-iron vegetables such as kale, spinach, and beets; and nourishing, grounding foods like sweet potatoes, pumpkin, peas, beans, okra, and carrots. If you are addicted to carbohydrates such as bread, pasta, and potatoes but put on weight, try eating lots of pumpkin. It's rich in vitamin A and tastes delicious fixed with minced raw garlic and a dash of turmeric powder and pumpkin pie spice.

An occasional meal of eggs or salmon—or some other fish rich in Omega 3 oils, such as mackerel, cod, or sardines—may help you feel grounded. Other high-animal-protein foods come with complications such as cholesterol and acids.

Stews and soups are always easier to digest than most other protein and carbohydrate combinations. The cooking blends flavors and energies of the foods. Add the following tonic herbs to soups if you need more energy:

> **1 teaspoon or 1 capsule ashwagandha powder**
> **1 small piece Chinese ginseng**
> **½ teaspoon clove powder (for sexual weakness,**
>   **or wheezing from asthma)**

## Herbs to build vitality

If you have weak digestion, hypoglycemia, or depression, follow each meal with 6 to 10 pills of Xiao Yao Wan, a Chinese digestive remedy containing ginger, mint, and blood-building herbs. (See mail-order sources in the Herbal Access section at the back of this book.)

After meals you can take an adrenal tonic if your digestion is otherwise not a problem. I recommend Sexoton, a Chinese patent remedy. These small pills contain blood-building herbs, including rehmannia, dioscorea, cornus, moutan bark, poria fungus, alisma, cinnamon, and aconite root, which treat shortness of breath, fatigue, backache, and diarrhea. A homemade substitute would be to eat raw juiced or steamed spinach, carrots, and beets, adding cinnamon, clove, and ginger.

Other adrenal tonics include those from health food stores such as capsules of damiana or combinations of several ginsengs, including Chinese, American, and Siberian.

Avoid combinations that add cayenne to nerve tonic herbs such as gotu kola or Siberian ginseng because the effect is too strong, a bit like pouring pepper on the brain. Also avoid using ma huang, a diaphoretic herb (makes you perspire), which was never intended to be used as a stimulant by traditional Chinese medicine.

## Remedies to calm the mind and ease the spirit

Winter offers a fine opportunity to withdraw into your healing space and rebuild your nerves and brain with herbs. I like to take lots of calcium. It is soothing. It is vital for healthy adrenal glands and essential for conversion of fat and sugar into energy. It helps heal physical and emotional wounds, fight infections, and prevent fatigue.

A favorite source of calcium, aside from whole grains, seaweed, and green vegetables, is oyster shell. In Chinatown, herbalists pound the shells into small pieces and add other blood-building herbs, such as those in Sexoton, which help in absorption. But you can find oyster-shell calcium in pill form almost anywhere.

I also like to take powdered pearl from Chinatown to calm nervousness and clear my skin. Add a dose of pearl powder to a little water and swallow it before bed or take Jing Xiang Oyster Shell and Pearl Capsules. You will feel as though you are the pearl within an oyster.

## Herb of the season: ashwagandha

Ashwagandha, an East Indian root similar to Chinese ginseng although not as heating, rebuilds nerves and strengthens muscles. Because of this, it is an excellent tonic for people who exhaust themselves with work, worry, or sexual excess. It renews sexual energy for those who are weak, because it builds vitality and blood.

I have recommended the powdered herb or capsules with much success for nerve illnesses such as multiple sclerosis, where nerve tissue has been damaged, creating problems of fatigue and poor sense of balance. In India the herb is recommended, cooked with rice, for expectant mothers who need to strengthen abdominal muscles and ease lower back pain.

Ashwagandha is a genuine tonic herb that generates health without creating nervousness. Since it is not "speed" but a nerve tonic, the herb will actually give a night of peaceful sleep to people who are too tired to rest. During that rest, vitality can be enhanced. As vigor is recovered, the herb will no longer be needed by the body to deepen sleep. Its tonic properties will come forth to engage the depths of our resilience and courage as muscles and bones feel young again.

Take capsules of ashwagandha after meals as needed. Start with one or two a day and increase the dosage as is comfortable, up to no more than four daily. One capsule equals ¼ teaspoon of the powder. Do not take this herb if your tongue is red, dry, or yellow-coated because it may be too heating. Instead, build moisture and sexual fluids with fo-ti, called he shou wu in Chinese. The dosage for this blood-building herb is usually five pills between meals three times daily. The Chinese pills are called Shou Wu Pien.

Ashwagandha capsules can be found in health food stores, and the powder is for sale in East Indian groceries. Shou Wu Pien, or dried sliced he shou wu, is available in Chinese herb shops and by mail order.

## The quick fix

For a fast boost to your stamina and enthusiasm, add a pinch of clove powder to a cup of hot water and drink it as tea. This kitchen spice works especially well during the late afternoon slump for people with pale tongues, weakness, and lethargy. It increases breathing for those with wheezing asthma and TB because it is a stimulant for lungs and adrenal energy.

# A Pleasure Cure

Cold weather and fatigue make us crave sweets. The pleasure cure for January, February, and any other time that you crave chocolate but do not want the calories is Chyavanprash. It may be spelled slightly differently when you find it in East Indian groceries, but it's pronounced "cha vahn prash." It is rich and delicious! Many people have given up eating chocolate after tasting this thick paste of ghee (clarified butter) and sweet kitchen spices.

Chyavanprash, an Ayurvedic medicine (from India), builds endurance and vitality because it contains tonic herbs, including ashwagandha and spices such as clove, cinnamon, cardamom, and many others. I like to spread it on toast for breakfast or as a snack. The dosage is only one or two tablespoons twice daily.

# Special Problems: Seasonal Depression and Insomnia

Do you suffer from sunshine deprivation during the winter? Around December, I am usually tempted to post a sign at home: "Take a bitch to the beach!" Warming herbs that step up metabolism can at least remind your body how nice warm weather feels.

Two warming herbal remedies are especially helpful in dreary weather because they treat depression. Contrary to popular scientific research, depression is not perceived by way of brain chemicals. Most people have absolutely no direct perception of their serotonin level. Instead, they feel heavy, logy, and off-center. Our emotional center is also our digestive center.

Xiao Yao Wan heals anxiety and depression with ginger, mint, and blood-building Chinese herbs that free stuck circulation. These pills are available in Chinese herb shops and supermarkets and by mail order from addresses found in the Herbal Access section at the back of this book. Use a dosage that suits you, anywhere from four to ten pills after meals or as needed. Xiao Yao Wan treats hypoglycemia, hiatal hernia, chest pain, and stress.

Kava kava is a pepper that treats depression by stimulating metabolism as it opens perception. This health food store capsule is recommended as a rejuvenator for people who are weak and who suffer from chills and the blahs. Avoid high doses of such warming tonics if you have frequent thirst, fever, or a dry red tongue. People with these overheated symptoms need cooler antidepression herbs such as a tea made by steeping a handful of dried Chinese red rosebuds.

If you have anxiety or insomnia during the winter months, you need to take something that will not decrease your vitality. One health food cure is Calms Forte, a homeopathic combination of herbs and minerals, including iron and calcium, that has been used for generations. The calming effect of the easily absorbed minerals will let you relax and sleep. You can melt a dose of these small pills in a cup of hot water at bedtime or any time you're nervous.

If you can't find this product, you might make your own version by combining one dose each of homeopathic ferrum phos. (iron), calc. phos. (calcium), nat. phos. (antiacid form of sodium), kali. phos. (potassium, a nerve tonic), and sedative herbs such as vervain, hops, or linden tea. If you can't sleep because of indigestion, try a cup of soothing catnip tea. (Share it with your cat.) It also treats colic.

Another effective way to ground yourself and sleep is a bedtime foot massage with raw sesame oil. Then wear cotton socks to bed. The last empress of China preferred to drink hot water to which was added a traditional nerve medicine—precious powdered pearl, another way to get your minerals. It comes in prepared tiny doses that you mix with a little spoon from Chinese herbal shops.

# In Your Healing Space

Winter is a time to pull inward to discover the richness of your interior life. You can make the most of this by spending time in your healing space. When I've taught rejuvenation workshops in the past, some students have gained a great deal by putting their baby picture into their healing space. Periodically, they would engage in a dialogue with the former self, discussing plans or disappointments in a way that comforted the child. We often lose touch with who is deep inside us. Sometimes we need to be reminded of what we really want before we can bound into the adventures of another spring. But don't stop there—in the sandbox with your inner child. Let's go beyond that.

## Visualization

When you were a child, what was your greatest ambition or desire? (I loved to dance and wanted to own a horse.) Visualize yourself with friends or alone expressing that desire. What of that desire has remained to this day? How can you adjust or satisfy the desire? Did the wish lead you to specific work, play, relationships, or travel? Do you still have the desire? Your childhood dream must be clarified and updated in order to be realized.

Children can be demanding and cruel. Inner children are no different. They want immediate satisfaction. They have no sense of reality. Be kind to yourself as you remember your childhood ambitions. It has taken a long time to develop the skills necessary to accomplish what you've done.

Using those skills to help others in some way will satisfy your inner child's demand for approval and love.

# Spring

In winter's dark stillness, the seeds of spring are born. The budding of life on earth is the dawn of new life in you. Use the springtime to begin new projects and directions. An ancient Chinese medical text advises movement in order to take advantage of spring's verdant power. We are told to rise early, let our hair fall loose, and walk briskly in the cool, damp air of the yard. We take this to mean that in spring we should bend, stretch, and use herbs that increase circulation. I dance and take bitter cleansers such as dandelion and tonics such as nettle.

## March, April, and May—Hope Springs Eternal

*Weather:* Cool, humid, windy, rainy, changeable; pollution

*Symptoms:* Nervous irritability, unstable emotions, headache, dizziness, aching joints, insomnia, water retention, congestion, allergies, spasms, or nerve illnesses

*Goals:* To cleanse liver and blood, to quiet nerves, and to follow anticancer and anticholesterol routines

*Supplies:* Dandelion, aloe, myrrh, green foods, alfalfa, nettle, wheat grass, cumin, coriander, fennel seeds, juniper berries, mint, dill, Wuchaseng, gotu kola

*Herb of the Season:* Dandelion

*The Quick Fix:* Homeopathic Natrum Sulphate 30c

*A Pleasure Cure:* A delicious chlorophyll drink

*Special Problems:* Allergic swelling—homeopathic apis mel. 30c; rage—aloe vera, Lung Tan Xie Gan Wan

Spring's rain and humidity require stimulating herbs that help the body to dissolve impurities. They may be laxatives and diuretics that treat water retention. Dandelion, parsley, juniper berries, red clover, aloe, and all sorts of bitter and sour salad greens speed elimination, clearing the body of excess weight and sluggishness. Often springtime allergies can be allayed by a strong liver-cleansing regime done weeks before allergy season. Spring winds may irritate the nerves with neuralgia, headaches, and muscle aches. Nervous irritability can lead to insomnia, anger, and frustration, all made worse by spicy hot foods, allergies, and spasm pain.

I strongly recommend avoiding job and home changes and especially arguments about money and divorce during the spring. The season's emotional irritations are often provoked by pollen irritants.

# Plan for the Season

Rid the body of acid conditions that underlie anger, depression, and pain. Teas that reduce cholesterol and antiacid foods are in order. Blood tonics that enhance sleep are helpful as are large doses of leafy greens, rich in chlorophyll, that soothe the nerves and build emotional resilience. Remember a green twig bends in the wind, but a dry old branch snaps. Oats and greens will make you limber, especially when cooked in water with a dash of turmeric.

## Spring teas

I could begin every diet recommendation of every month of the year with green tea, but especially in spring. Try to start the day with a pot of green tea because it reduces weight, water retention, and cholesterol. If you are still addicted to coffee and suffer headaches from withdrawal, add a dose of homeopathic belladonna 30c to your green tea. The homeopathic remedy treats fever and hot, throbbing pains such as withdrawal headaches.

Other useful teas are made of catnip, a digestive, and of sedative herbs such as vervain, linden, rosebud, mint, and valerian root.

## Spring foods

Cooling, moistening foods such as oats, rice, seeds, almonds, tofu, and all sorts of fruits and vegetables will be helpful. Dairy foods will feel especially congesting in spring and autumn. Instead, add rice or soy milk to cereals. Simply adding one or two meals of these foods daily to your regular diet will eventually improve your circulation and mood.

I often make fresh green salads, combining digestive herbs such as mint, parsley, raw fennel root (anise), dill, coriander leaf, and cabbage. I make the dressing with raw ginger, tamari, olive oil, a few drops of sesame oil, lemon juice, and balsamic vinegar in which I've steeped fresh tarragon for a couple of weeks.

## Herbs for water retention

Stimulant diuretic herbs such as dandelion, sarsaparilla, and juniper berries can help eliminate water buildup. Vitamin $B_6$ helps, as do apple cider vinegar and lecithin.

Chinese doctors recommend fu-ling, a white fungus, harvested from around the roots of certain trees. You can boil a handful of dried fu-ling in two cups of water for twenty minutes to make a decoction that relieves difficult urination. Recommended for persons with a thickly coated tongue, this tea helps clear the urine of deposits that may form stones. Other diuretic formulas available in health food stores will be covered in Chapter 9.

## Headache and dizziness

Valerian is recommended for nerve-related headache pain, migraine, and dizziness. You know it's a nervous headache when all you want to do is lie down in a dark room and turn off the phone. You crave isolation because your nerves are overstimulated. I also use a capsule of valerian for in-flight airplane headaches due to noise, excitement, and air conditioning.

## Joint aches and backache

Luckily, a number of excellent American-manufactured brands exist to treat arthritis or stiff joints. Among them are homeopathic rhus tox. 6x or 30c. If you use 6x strength, take a dose five times daily for chronic stiffness and pain that feels better with warmth and movement. If the pain is acute, use the 30c strength.

ArthPlus, made by Nature's Herbs, contains many of the major herbs used to treat painful joints—yucca, white willow bark, hydrangea root, devil's claw, alfalfa leaves, burdock, black cohosh root, sarsaparilla, prickly ash bark, slippery elm bark, cayenne, licorice root, parsley root and leaves, along with trace minerals. This type of combination hits all bases—it contains cleansing herbs, natural pain relievers, hormonal precursors (cohosh and sarsaparilla), and nutritive tonics (alfalfa and trace minerals).

Sometimes it's nice to have something special to rub onto your aching back. Chinese analgesic patches contain as many as seventy stimulant herbs on a sticky tape you can put directly on your skin. These patches are fun but messy. They also leave a sting or stain on your skin for days. A better option is a rub-in cream or oil, either Tiger Balm, medicated wintergreen oil, or a new import from India, Boswellin Cream (from *Boswellia serrata,* similar to frankincense) made by Nature's Herbs. The fragrance is mild and the warmth penetrates deep to help ease spasm.

## Herbs to soothe the brain and nerves

Some people think too much. New Yorkers are especially guilty. It makes them nervous and jumpy. Aside from a nice trip to the Caribbean, one way to ease tension and improve brain function if you are fried from overwork is to take a nerve tonic such as gotu kola. This Himalayan rejuvenation herb improves memory, decreases aging and senility, and fortifies the adrenal glands. When you take it regularly you almost feel as though your brain can finally take a deep breath and relax. It's not a sedative, but helps both brain hemispheres work in better coordination.

Take six capsules of gotu kola throughout the day for smooth, steady energy and sweet nighttime sleep. If you are anxious, combine gotu kola with Wuchaseng, a Chinese extract of Siberian ginseng that is particularly suited to calm nerves. Stronger dosages of this herb are stimulants used by athletes for increased energy. You can calm and collect yourself before bed by preparing a tea made of one teaspoon of the Chinese liquid extract added to a cup of hot water. Take this along with two capsules of gotu kola for a brain vacation.

## Herb of the season: dandelion

Springtime's herb is dandelion, the all-powerful cleanser. It dissolves excess acid, fibroids, gallstones, and fat, with laxative and diuretic action. The trick is to take a lot of it. Treat it like a salad in a capsule and swallow handfuls throughout the day. Dandelion is full of useful vitamins and minerals. Other sources of cleansing-building nutrients can be found in nettle and alfalfa.

## The quick fix

If you feel nauseated and dizzy from pollution or from eating the wrong foods, take a dose or two of homeopathic nat. sulph. 30c, a liver cleanser. It will also clear jaundiced facial coloring, asthma made worse by excess humidity, and bad breath brought on by eating too many fatty foods.

# A Pleasure Cure

Liquid chlorophyll makes such a delicious sweet drink that you may want to add the bottled version to sparkling water as a refreshing drink. It makes you feel as though you've swallowed the lawn. It freshens your breath, skin, and eyes so that you feel all new. I pour about ⅛ cup or more into a large wineglass of water. It turns your elimination chartreuse.

# Special Problems: Allergic Swelling and Rage

Some people puff up with mean allergic swellings from cosmetics, airborne irritants, or pollens. The swelling can be red-hot, like bee stings. Certain foods can make the throat swell closed to cause suffocation. If your allergic reactions involve such swelling, take a dose or two of homeopathic apis mel. 30c (homeopathic honey bee) to counter bee-sting type irritations. The swelling will resolve, usually within one half hour. During allergy season, carry this remedy with you when you're near allergens.

Rage is not limited to spring, but it can be worse when tempers are high from nerve irritants, allergens, and all sorts of people suffering from aches and pains. Instead of avoiding all social contacts, quiet your nerves directly with aloe vera gel. This health food store version of magic salve is usually spread on the skin to heal wounds and burns, or drunk for ulcers, but the cure for rage is to put aloe gel into your nose.

The nose has blood vessels and nerves that communicate directly with the brain. Putting aloe vera gel into your nose with a Q-Tip or dropper is like dousing a brain fire with clear Jell-O. It soothes fretting and fuming as it relaxes your nerves.

In China a pill remedy called Lung Tan Xie Gan Wan is used in large doses—thirty or more little black pills daily—to reduce anger and violent behavior. It soothes headache, constipation, and herpes with gentle digestive herbs that cleanse the liver and gallbladder. The normal dose is somewhere between twelve and twenty pills taken throughout the day.

A Western herbal equivalent might be one-quarter cup of aloe vera gel added daily to apple juice along with ten drops each of gentian, burdock root, and sarsaparilla extracts. This juice can be taken all day between meals. The effect is cooling and balancing for liverish symptoms.

According to traditional Chinese medicine, when the wood element is healthy, we can easily make and carry out decisions. This is partly because if the liver is healthy, we can absorb calcium, which is necessary for strength, elasticity, and calm. Spring can derange the wood element to the point where physical and emotional strength and elasticity are lost. We struggle to stay calm or change directions, when our "wood" has turned to sawdust, but green foods, rich in calcium, keep us young and fresh.

# In Your Healing Space

Spring energy embraces the high vitality of change, movement, and flowering. Bring a green plant into your healing space. Honor yourself as though you were a green plant—with plenty of sunlight, water, and fresh air. Turn to page 157 to find recipes for wonderful raw vegetable juices. Use your healing space to stretch, do yoga or tai chi, to dance, or to have a massage.

Use fresh scents as body rubs and incense such as evergreen, patchouli, clover, green apple, or any other light, spicy fragrance.

Scrub your body with a paste made of sea salt, baking soda, and water. Shower off, and then apply this seaweed beauty pack for toning the skin, which reduces cellulite.

### Seaweed Pack

**1 cup plain instant oatmeal**
**2 ounces dulce seaweed (soaked until soft)**
**2 ounces laminaria seaweed (soaked until soft)**
**Corn oil and nat. sulph. 6x**

Simmer the oatmeal a few minutes, until it is soft but not runny. Add the seaweed and whip the mixture in a blender until it is smooth but not liquid. Or add ten crushed Laminaria 4 pills. Add a dose of nat. sulph. 6x to a tablespoon of corn oil. Add enough oil to make a sticky paste.

Apply this warm to clean dry skin. Let it become dry before you remove it with wet paper towels. Follow with a cool shower.

### Activity

What will you do with your springtime excess energy? Taking cooling, cleansing herbs has its limits. Try doing something that you've never done before, something physical you've always wanted to do. It may be related to your unaccomplished desire, the visualization found on page 72, or it may be completely different. If you're totally at a loss for what to do, ask the *I Ching* for advice. You may enjoy doing artwork, or you could make something that involves your time, energy, and spirit, then offer it to someone as a gift.

# Summer

With the full bloom of summer at hand, we must protect ourselves from heat and dehydration with cooling, moistening, and cleansing herbs. Some are delicious teas we can share with friends.

## June, July, and August—Summer Flowers

*Weather:* Hot, hazy; pollution
*Symptoms:* Fever, heat stroke, thirst, excitability

*Goals:* To cool and cleanse the body and to follow an anticancer
routine

*Supplies:* Honeysuckle flower, dandelion, sarsaparilla, American
ginseng tea

*Herb of the Season:* American ginseng tea

*The Quick Fix:* Homeopathic belladonna 30c

*A Pleasure Cure:* Chinese chrysanthemum tea

*Special Problems:* Hot flashes—skullcap, Shou Wu Pien;
eczema—honeysuckle-dandelion tea

I remember the sound of crickets and the heavy sweetness of honeysuckle flowers outside my window as a child. Summer nights, we'd lie
awake unable to move under the weight of the honeysuckle's fragrance.
Days, our work was clearing the flower beds of dandelions. Mother
loved her roses and collected ever more delicate hues, but my herbalist
grandmother's stinky snapdragons, dahlias, marigolds, and mums were
her pride. Many flowers are potent healing herbs. Marigold tea is recommended for ulcers, cramps, and diarrhea. You can dry them from
your garden or order them from herb shops listed in the Herbal Access
section.

Summer's heat can cause problems such as heat stroke, thirst, dry
skin, and weakness. Cooling, moistening herbs will help, but you may also
need to cleanse impurities and excess acids.

# Plan for the Season

Use summer's heat and the perspiration it causes to your advantage. By
adding cleansing herbs and homeopathic remedies to your diet, you can
help rid your body of fat and fibroids. Sweating is very important. Some
researchers say that women who vigorously exercise regularly reduce
their risk of breast cancer, although the researchers are not sure why. It
may be, at least in part, the sweating that helps dissolve masses. We lose
weight and impurities by sweating. Summer offers an excellent opportunity for it.

## Summer teas

Cooling drinks can be made by adding a dash of any of the following digestive yet relaxing spices to a non-caffeine tea: cumin, fennel, coriander
seeds or powder, or fresh mint. To soothe acid indigestion and eliminate
bad breath, add a handful of fresh parsley and up to one-quarter cup of
aloe juice or gel to tea or juice.

## Summer foods

You will suffer less from summer's heat if you add the following cooling
foods to your regular diet: all sorts of berries and cherries, basmati white
rice, rice milk, tofu, steamed greens, laxative foods such as squashes,
green beans, salads, almonds, seeds, vegetable and wheat grass juices.

## Herbs for rich eating and drinking

In summer we are often tempted to eat richly and too late at night to easily digest. It's wonderful to linger in cafés, eating and drinking with
friends. Here are some ways to celebrate without suffering.

After eating and drinking too much, causing digestive pain, headache,
hangover, or crabbiness, take a couple of doses of homeopathic nux. vomica
30c, made from a bitter nut. It works for hangovers, too.

## Honeysuckle for sore throat and blemishes

Honeysuckle flower tea is useful if you have a cold with a sore throat and
fever any time of year because it is a cooling broad-spectrum antibiotic
that works specifically on throat, lungs, large intestine, and skin. Medical
research has shown that it inhibits in vitro growth of salmonella,
Staphylococcus aureus, Streptococcus pneumoniae, tuberculosis, and influenza.
In China it has also been used for appendicitis, chronic conjunctivitis, and
corneal ulcers. Honeysuckle is always an ingredient in skin blemish pill
remedies from China.

For fever and sore throat, simmer a handful of dried honeysuckle flowers in a liter of water for twenty minutes and drink one to three cups daily.

It can be laxative in higher doses. For itchy rashes including eczema, add a handful of dandelion herb to the honeysuckle flowers and simmer as above.

## A healing diuretic

You may need a diuretic in the summer because urination is reduced when we perspire more than usual. Sarsaparilla tea is a diuretic that contains valuable hormones that benefit both men and women. It was traditionally used to soothe burning urination and treat sexually transmitted disease. More recently it has been used to reduce water retention, dark, cloudy urine, and prostate discomfort. East Indian (Ayurvedic) doctors feel that drinking sarsaparilla tea regularly reduces negative emotions, which goes to show just how irritating excess acids can become.

You can empty one or two sarsaparilla capsules into a cup of tea and drink it after meals, but not before bed.

## Herb of the season: American ginseng

American ginseng, either the instant tea or the tea made from the root, can be used to replace needed moisture during hot weather. It increases saliva and softens the skin. Its action is the opposite of Chinese or Korean red ginseng, which are both high-energy tonics. American ginseng is a different plant altogether. Take it after you've had a fever, if you have hot flashes, or if you are often thirsty. If you are using the sliced root, simmer a handful in a liter of spring water for twenty minutes and drink a cup or more a day.

Do not use American ginseng if you have chills, a cold, or asthma unless you have a dry cough. It makes more moisture and therefore more congestion at those times.

## The quick fix

Homeopathic belladonna 30c is great for when you get a sudden hot, throbbing headache from the weather, from a fever, or from eating the wrong thing. It cools liverish anger, but is used most often for hot, burning physical symptoms. I recommend it for people who want to stop drinking coffee but who suffer from withdrawal headaches.

# A Pleasure Cure

For pure delight and a relaxing, healing drink for your eyes, brew a pinch of Chinese chrysanthemum flowers as a pot of tea. They are delicious—sweet as honey, only better. They are recommended for eyestrain, cloudy vision, and headache. You can order them from Chinese herb shops listed in the Herbal Access section at the back of the book. Add the dried flowers to a transparent glass teapot, because when you add boiling water, the flowers expand.

# Special Problems: Hot Flashes and Insomnia

Although there is no particular season for hot flashes or insomnia, you'll feel them both worse from summer heat and excess caffeine. First stop drinking coffee. Try green tea, adding homeopathic belladonna 30c if you get withdrawal symptoms.

Skullcap herb is very effective for cooling anger, hot flashes, and insomnia due to liverish irritation from eating spicy foods or any other reason. For calming relief, add ten to twenty drops of skullcap extract to a wineglass of spring water or take two capsules before bed.

Summer is a good time to take anticancer herbs; they can become part of your weight-loss or cleansing routine. See my recommendations beginning on page 131.

# In Your Healing Space

Summer is a good time to be social, to travel, and to sweat, according to an ancient Chinese medical text. Break through your limits at the gym. Go beyond your norm with dance or movement, and stretch your intellectual horizons by attending concerts, plays, and other performances.

## Emotional clearing

Do you want to try new things, but hear a little voice in your head saying, "But that's not so easy. That's not *you*. *You* can't do that!"?

You can break through emotional blocks that trip up your original you by stimulating vitality. Movement not only gets your endorphins (natural painkillers) going; it can also break apart old patterns of every sort. Stuck circulation keeps your thoughts about everything going through the same energy channels.

You hold memories in your body. When you move, sweat, and stretch beyond your usual limits, you break through to another part of yourself, to uncharted experience, perhaps even a former life. I think we were all animals and plants before we got a chance to be human. Remember the bird you once were. Birds can fly anywhere they want without getting advanced college degrees or corporate jobs.

A traditional remedy for obsession, which can be no more than stuck ideas, is to drink cinnamon tea. Add one-half teaspoon cinnamon powder per cup. It will make you perspire and at the same time will unglue stagnant energy patterns.

If you have excess thirst, feverish conditions, or hot flashes, add one pinch cinnamon to American ginseng tea, the cooling, moistening type of ginseng.

# Autumn

Use this invigorating time of year to set yourself straight: weed out the closets, patch up old grudges, and drop lethargy as you clear your mucus.

## September, October, November, and December—Harvest

*Weather:* Cold, dry, rain, snow, artificial heat

*Symptoms:* Fatigue, stiffness, chills, colds, flu, depression, sexual weakness, overwork, poor memory

*Goals:* To prevent colds, flu, asthma, and pain; to maintain high energy; to clear blemishes; and to prevent depression

*Supplies:* Pungent foods (radish, parsley, carrot); stimulating spices (clove, ginger); tonic herbs (astragalus, epimedium); herbs that clear blemishes (Herba Oldenlandia Diffusa Beverage)

*Herb of the Season:* Astragalus

*The Quick Fix:* Homeopathic pulsatilla 30c

*A Pleasure Cure:* Osha brandy

*Special Problems:* Skin blemishes—antibiotic herbs, including Lien Chiao Pai Tu Pien; depression—rosebud tea, Xiao Yao Wan, Co-schizandra Tablets

Autumn and winter are hard times for people who have difficulty breathing. Inhalation can become shallow from fatigue and cold weather. We require more vital energy during cold weather for immune strength and courage. This is because when we are tired or as a reaction to cold, our energy draws inward to protect our internal organs. This season's foods should be warm, nourishing, stimulating, and in some cases, diaphoretic (making us perspire).

# Plan for the Season

Foods and herbs that are sweet and pungent stimulate energy—for example, grains cooked with clove, ginger, and cinnamon. Sweet, heavy foods and oils sedate the nerves and are useful for insomnia—for example, sweet potato seasoned with olive oil and nutmeg. East Indian doctors cook nerve tonic herbs along with milk gruel to ensure nourishment and endurance, but this is not practical or palatable for most Americans. Instead, spend the fall and winter making delicious soups and stews, adding the right kinds of tonic herbs.

## Autumn teas

Use these herbs to make pleasant teas that increase sweating. They are best used to prevent hypothermia after you have come inside for the day. Steep one pinch of pungent herb per cup, using one of the following: cinnamon, basil, raw ginger, or honeysuckle and chrysanthemum flower instant tea. The spices are from the supermarket and the prepared Chinese tea is available by mail or in Chinese groceries.

## Autumn foods

If you and your family are often weak and chilled, use invigorating herbs such as Chinese ginseng and tang kuei, a warming blood-building herb, when making chicken or vegetable soup. If you have tired, weak legs and low sexual energy, make a tea using aphrodisiac herbs such as *Epimedium grandiflorum* (yin yang huo). Simmer a handful of the leaves for twenty minutes and pour the mild-tasting liquid over tea leaves or drink it plain. Epimedium is an adrenal tonic herb that also protects the heart.

## Herbs to prevent and treat colds and flu

If you frequently catch cold, you will need to use a lot of herbs that help sweat out the cold such as teas made with ginger, scallions, and cinnamon. Remember, herbs and nutrients used to prevent colds, such as vitamin C, zinc, or garlic, will not help you after you catch a cold. You'll have to sweat it out. You will enjoy making and drinking osha brandy (page 129) to protect your lungs and vital energy from the cold.

## Herbs for nervous conditions

If you have trouble sleeping or are racked with nerve pains, the earthy fragrant herb valerian, a nerve sedative, can be helpful. Swallow one or two capsules for nerve pain, nervous insomnia, or migraine as needed.

## Herb of the season: astragalus

Astragalus is a Chinese herb that we are beginning to hear a great deal about and see quite often in American herbal pharmacies. In China it is used as a major health food to build immunity to colds, allergies, and even cancer. It stops excessive sweating resulting from weakness, fatigue, and water retention. You can find capsules made by American manufacturers in health food stores. If you are weak and run-down or if you fear or have had cancer, take six to eight capsules daily before cold and allergy season—usually sometime in early autumn. If you are boiling the dried herb slices, simmer one handful of astragalus in a liter of spring water for at least twenty minutes and drink the liquid as tea or soup stock daily.

## The quick fix

Dreary weather can make you feel blue. If you can't stop weeping and have difficulty breathing from thick mucus, take homeopathic pulsatilla 30c. It clears congestion and lifts the emotional fog. Add a dose to a cup of hot water and sip it throughout the day. After the fog has lifted, you can take a dose five times a day, or as needed. Remember, when taking homeopathic remedies, do not mix them with food, drink, or toothpaste. The best times to take them are first thing in the morning, one-half hour before eating or two hours after eating. But in emergencies or during a long-term weepy depression, take homeopathic pulsatilla throughout the entire day.

## A Pleasure Cure

Chilly weather wears down resistance so that you may feel weak after being outside. To prevent colds and flu, hypothermia, or depression, make a delicious healing beverage—actually an herbal tincture—that clears lungs and sinus of mucus.

Osha grows wild in the American Southwest at elevations above 9,000 feet. I don't try to harvest it myself because it too closely resembles fool's parsley, which is dangerous. You can buy or order dried osha root from herb shops, but I like to get mine directly from Sabinita, the herbalist in Truchas, New Mexico.

For clearing the lungs and sweating out the cold, we use the osha root rather than the plant. Its aroma is pungent-sweet, a bit like brandy. That gave me the idea to make a tincture—an alcohol extract—using brandy: Steep an osha root in a bottle of brandy for three weeks and use the resulting brew sparingly, ten to twenty drops at a time in a little water. Drink it one half hour after meals or before going to bed because it may make you perspire. The diaphoretic (sweating) action works to clear congestion. Osha is more pleasant and less harmful to use than echinacea because it is not an antibiotic. Osha can be used every day. Unlike echinacea, it will not make you feel overheated and dizzy, nor will it disrupt digestion.

Echinacea is a harsh, drying, and inflammatory herb that I do not recommend using for longer than a day at a time. Many people now are taking echinacea and goldenseal daily during cold and flu season. Although they are both strong antibiotic herbs—echinacea works best for upper respiratory tract infections and goldenseal for yeast and infections in the lower gastrointestinal tract—they can be irritating and draining.

Echinacea makes you perspire and, for that reason, is too drying. Never use it with a dry cough or fever. It causes dizziness when used to excess. After a week or two of echinacea and goldenseal you can expect a dry cough, rough skin, bloating, indigestion, and possibly anxiety. If you want to use something less irritating than echinacea to build up your immunity against colds and flu, use astragalus.

# Special Problems: Skin Blemishes and Depression

Complexion problems are one of the complications of this season of reduced light and oxygen. When we are tired and eat rich foods, our body has less chance to digest. Impurities can end up affecting the skin. We need to step up cleansing when digestion and breathing are impaired.

Most Asian herbal formulas that treat skin problems contain at least one antibiotic herb and one blood or liver cleanser. The simplest is Xiao Yan Sanjie Tablets (*Senecionis scandentis*). Other more complicated pills from Chinatown's herb stores include Lien Chiao Pai Tu Pien, which combines honeysuckle; antifever herbs such as forsythia bark, gardenia bud, and skullcap; and digestive remedies, including orange peel, caraway seed, and rhubarb. Take four pills three times daily or as needed. Avoid fried, hot, spicy, or creamy rich foods and sugar.

Depression is another result of reduced vitality and impaired blood production. It is true that depression has no season, but many people feel it more during cold gray days. The reduced light affects the production of brain chemicals such as serotonin, a mood stabilizer. They say that daylight and an ocean setting are particularly good for stimulating the brain's uptake of serotonin. But the scientists do not wonder what else is affected. At the beach and in pleasant weather, we breathe deeper and digest better because we are relaxed.

Certain digestive herbs work well to clear sinus congestion, improve breathing, and enhance digestion. When depressed we feel heavy, weary, hopeless. It's like being adrift on a sea of troubles. However, improving digestion can enforce our sense of being centered and grounded: we feel more at home in our body.

Xiao Yao Wan is a Chinese pill formula that brings us back to our digestive center. Its herbs, including ginger, mint, bupleurum, tang kuei, atractylodes, paeonia, and poria, help balance blood sugar, ease chest pain, and reduce tension. It contains digestive and blood-building herbs that ensure vitality and mental clarity. There is no one correct dosage for such an herbal formula. It would be like advising you to eat a certain amount of food. If you have hypoglycemia or feel weak, chilled, and have a pale tongue, you may need to take a handful of these small pills three or more times a day. You may also want to add other fortifying stimulant herbs to your soups—ginger, mint, tarragon, parsley, rosemary, sage, or spinach, for example.

## In Your Healing Space

For an afternoon lift that helps clear your head and reduce chest discomfort, brew a handful of dried Chinese red rosebuds as a pot of tea. They have been recommended for depression, headache, and generally feeling out of sorts. Sold in Chinese herb shops, they are used not for making potpourri but for making tea. Another nice flower tea is made of dried lavender flowers. Their spicy aroma lifts your spirits.

### A gift of love

Throughout the year in your healing space you have reconnected with your inner child, not to mention your inner frog, fish, and bird. You have become the pearl within your inner oyster. You have stretched, danced, and conceived of and carried out new projects. Now, during autumn and winter harvest, take stock of your year and share hopes and plans with someone. You may write a love note or a job proposal, but put your heart, mind, and energy into it. Your work to help alleviate others' suffering will open many doors to your spiritual awakening.

## Cancer: Extra-Strong Prevention

You can feel confident about using any of my recommendations for the seasons because they are just exaggerated good sense. My herbal advice contains a level of sophistication beyond folk remedies because it's based on traditional Asian medicine. Certain ailments are expected to happen at certain times and in predictable ways. The patterns are set down by nature. Traditional Asian medicine studies how nature makes her invisible life force manifest with changes in the seasons.

The fear of illness threatens vitality and concentration. It's better to use a *treatment*—not just a preventive measure—than to wait with white knuckles for disease to strike. That's why I take stronger-than-usual herbs at various times of the year to prevent (and treat) heart disease and fibroids. Traditional Asian medicine provides herbal remedies that safely dissolve impurities without harming the body or lowering vitality. They actually improve circulation while eliminating wastes and fat. Among them are antitumor herbs.

"Fibroid" and "tumor" are general terms in Asian medicine. They can mean anything from a lump in your breast to a superficial cyst or a malignant tumor. The approach used for their prevention is cleansing—that is, dissolving impurities such as excess acids and masses. Cleansing is a major part of prevention of most serious chronic illness. Our natural ability to cleanse is lessened by fatigue, stress, pollution, poor habits, and emotional imbalance. Fibroid prevention remedies stimulate natural cleansing processes. They increase circulation, enhance metabolism, and rid the body of wastes.

Here is something you did not know: you can take a smaller than usual dose of Chinese anticancer herbs regularly as part of a prevention program. These herbs do not weaken the body because we all benefit from cleansing. The following prevention remedies do not act on the cells like chemotherapy: they are cleansers, not destroyers. Directions are most often inside the box in English. If not, ask your herbalist to assist you.

According to traditional Asian diagnosis, if you feel weak and have a pale puffy tongue and a slow pulse, you require additional warming foods and tonic herbs such as Chinese ginseng and astragalus, taken during cleansing and prevention. If your tongue is red, dry, and cracked; if your pulse is fast and high; if you have fevers, night sweats, or high blood pressure, you will require additional cooling, moistening foods and herbs such as American ginseng or antifever herbs.

# Fibroid-Prevention Potions, Pills, and Capsules

This section offers a range of fibroid-prevention remedies—everything from teas you prepare at home to Chinese patent remedies available by mail order. Feel free to explore and choose from among them based on your predisposition and fears. They are safe, tested by time or in studies done in Chinese hospitals, and effective, for at least reducing the tendency to have tumors and the size of tumors. You can combine these remedies with nutritional programs. They can be used before or along with chemotherapy.

Chinese anti-fibroid herbal pills or capsules often contain animal products such as powdered musk, centipede, leech, or anteater scales. One popular capsule for prevention of breast and uterine fibroids even uses processed flying squirrel excrement. Tiny amounts of such animal products are used to greatly stimulate circulation in order to dissolve hard masses. If you prefer using only plant products, ask your herbalist to mix up an individual formula for you.

## Simple At-Home Prevention

My favorite remedies are often very simple and easily available from health food stores. For example, to promote deep internal cleansing, add up to one-quarter cup of aloe vera gel to water. Drink this once daily along with five capsules of dandelion and one of myrrh. This recipe combines two blood- and liver-cleansing herbs with one antitumor herb (myrrh). You may need to vary it according to your digestion. If you need more warmth and better circulation, use less aloe and more myrrh. If you need more laxative action, use more aloe and dandelion.

## Chinese Patent Formula Pills According to Fibroid Type

The herbal contents in Latin and English, the action of the herbs, and the dosage are printed on a separate sheet inside most boxes. Often extensive hospital research studies are cited, but you can find out even more by using the Internet. Look up the herbs and studies cited through Medline using Latin herbal names.

## Breast and uterine fibroids

According to the American Cancer Society, China has the lowest rate of breast cancer mortality in the world. This is certainly not due to lack of stress, pollution, or poor diet. Chinese women suffer plenty of stress, although, as a rule, they neither drink much nor smoke. Neither is their country's stunning success related to the use of mammograms, Western drug therapy, or surgery, all of which are too expensive to be used by the general population. Chinese herbs have traditionally been used to dissolve tumors for many generations. They really work.

Strong Xiao Jin Tan is recommended for prevention and treatment of breast and uterine fibroids. These are little red-and-yellow capsules that contain powdered herbs, including myrrh, musk, and a trace of dried flying squirrel dung. Traditional Chinese herbalists, like homeopathic physicians, believe that a trace of poison prompts the body to cleanse impurities. I use this formula regularly to eliminate breast fibroids and discomfort. The normal dosage is one pill twice daily. The higher dose for more serious cases, including cancer, is two pills twice a day. I combine it sometimes with dandelion capsules to make it work even more specifically for the breast. It can be used with no side effects between periods.

## Lung, cervical, and stomach tumors, and moles

Lian Bai Tablets have been proved "eminently effective against epithelioma villosum, cervical cancer, nasopharyngeal cancer, lung cancer, pharyngo cancer, stomach cancer and other cancerous diseases," according to the label. It is not unusual for such an anti-fibroid pill to be used for many different kinds of tumors, because the herbs cleanse more than one specific area of the body.

This pill contains rock arborvitae, gecko lizard, ophidia grass, prunella vulgaris, gallstone powder (probably from cows), musk, and "seven-leaf single branch flower." Someday in the best of all possible worlds of medical research, different nations will cooperate on testing these substances and will use the same nomenclature. For now I prefer to trust what is successful even if it is foreign. I have used this 2 to 4 pills daily for cleansing and have recommended it for people with fibroids, and all have reported greater energy and vitality.

## The works

Anticancerlin Sugar-coated Tablets from Shanghai Pharmaceutical Industry Corporation are sugar-coated pink pills used to treat malignant tumors. According to the directions printed inside the box in English, French, and Chinese, these pills rarely have side effects and can be used over the long term to reduce tumors, jaundice, and pain. They also improve appetite and vitality. The ingredients are part chemical and part herbal. Indicated chiefly for pancreatic, gastric, rectal, liver, and esophageal fibroids, but also for lung, urinary, bladder, nasopharyngeal, thyroid fibroids, and leukemia, the pills can be used after surgery to prolong remission time and build resistance. No digestive side effects such as nausea or diarrhea were reported when this cancer drug was extensively tested in Chinese hospitals.

I have personally used Anticancerlin taken along with Strong Xiao Jin Tan to great advantage. The powerful cleansing action of the two makes you feel as though breast lumps are dissolving before your very eyes.

# Long-Term Benefits of Prevention

Many people work and worry all the time. They eat poorly and on the run. They exercise little and are sure they will pay for it someday. The best way to avoid illness and paranoia is to take any of the above prevention remedies yearly for one or more months at a time, along with a sane cleansing diet of fruits, vegetables, grains, seeds, legumes, tofu, olive oil, raw vegetable juices, and green tea. Diabetic persons should avoid all sugars, including sweet vegetables such as beets. For those who still smoke, I recommend buying expensive life insurance.

I'm sometimes asked, "Can you go overboard with cleansing?" It is wise to alternately cleanse and build strength. You will be able to tell how much you should cleanse by observing your energy, mood, and symptoms. If you become weak, scattered, depressed, or chilled from cleansing, stop for a while and take an energy tonic that works well for you. If your tongue is severely coated with white, gray, brown, or green mucus, continue to cleanse with digestive and laxative herbs and foods.

Cleansing diets will make you look and feel wonderfully light and clean, but the total answer goes deeper than the surface. I once met a man who cleansed his body with raw juices five times daily for half the year. He drank enormous amounts of water and avoided all dietary impurities. This regime sounded extremely healthy, and he reported that it gave him tremendous energy and stamina. He looked a bit flushed, acted agitated, and occasionally pined for former bad habits. He could have benefited from energy-balancing or acupuncture to change the course of his cravings.

He was inflexible about his lifestyle to the point of having no time for anything else. Probably his health would have been much worse without all that cleansing, but his lifestyle made a normal life impossible. He lived with over fifty animals he'd collected from around the neighborhood only so he could have them spayed. He seemed the kind of guy who, if he wasn't watching his diet all the time, might have been an ax murderer.

I was reminded of something one of my favorite mentors, Dr. Bernard Jensen, once said: "Even if a man cleanses toxins all day long, if he doesn't have love in his heart, what kind of a husband can he make?" I think that goes for both sexes.

## Your five-day plan for winter or cold weather

*Morning:* Hot green tea with ½ teaspoon ashwagandha powder or ginger; cooked cereal with cinnamon, clove, orange peel, almonds, and vanilla

*Lunch and dinner:* Warm cooked foods, including kale, spinach, yams, tofu, root vegetables; warm digestive and stimulant spices; sage, fenugreek, rosemary, basil, clove, or cinnamon and turmeric; green or oolong tea

*Bedtime:* Warm soy milk with turmeric; Calms Forte or homeopathic ferrum phos. 6x, calc. phos. 6x, kali. phos. 6x

*Herbs:* Ginger, Chinese ginseng, Xiao Yao Wan, kava kava, hawthorn

## Your five-day plan for spring or humid weather

*Morning:* Hot green tea with fresh mint or dandelion coffee substitute; oatmeal and soy or rice milk with cumin, coriander, and fennel powder.

*Lunch and dinner:* Cooling nourishing foods including salads and cooked green vegetables, seaweeds, radishes, onions, red cabbage, cucumbers, fresh fennel, tarragon, mint, dill, cilantro; liquid chlorophyll drink

*Bedtime:* Aloe vera in apple juice or homeopathic nat. sulph. 6x; gotu kola

*Herbs:* Dandelion, honeysuckle, alfalfa, yucca, corn silk, nettle, and red clover capsules; gentian extract or digestive bitters in water after meals

## Your five-day plan for summer or hot weather

*Morning:* Hot green tea with a dash of digestive bitters; American ginseng; fresh fruit only or vegetables with toast, cereal, or fish

*Lunch and dinner:* Fresh fruits or vegetables, salads, and clean proteins such as tofu and tempeh; Chinese chrysanthemum tea or skullcap extract; nat. sulph. 6x (dizziness, nausea) or homeopathic belladonna 30c for heatstroke

*Bedtime:* apple or cool green drink of fresh vegetables

*Herbs:* Anti-fibroid herbs, aloe, and myrrh

## Your five-day plan for autumn or cool and dry weather

*Morning:* Hot green tea and hot spices, radishes; sprout bread, scallions, ginger; dried fruits, including apricots; grape-seed extract

*Lunch and dinner:* Warm, nourishing low-fat foods and stimulant spices; anti-candida diet and Australian Tea Tree Oil tea

*Herbs:* Astragalus, 6 capsules daily; cold-prevention herbs; homeopathic pulsatilla 30c for mucus and depression as needed

# Keys

*Winter*—Mixed trace minerals, Chinese ginseng, fo-ti
    Warming: Cinnamon, clove, ginger, or basil tea
    Depression: Kava kava capsules, rosebud tea, homeopathic
       pulsatilla, homeopathic gelsemium, homeopathic aconite

*Spring*—Homeopathic nat. sulph. 30c, nettle
    Cleansing: Dandelion, aloe vera, mint, alfalfa, cornsilk tea

*Summer*—Aloe vera, myrrh, American ginseng
    Cooling for heatstroke: Homeopathic belladonna 30c

*Autumn*—Astragalus, dang shen
    Colds and flu: Gan Mao Ling, basil, honeysuckle, thyme

**Links:** Also see Chapters 3, 8, 12, 13, 16

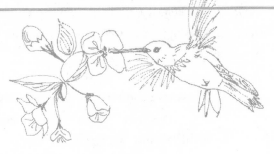

# PART THREE

# ETERNAL YOUTH

*The life force within you is nameless,
shapeless, and electric. It lasts forever.
It is your personal miracle.*

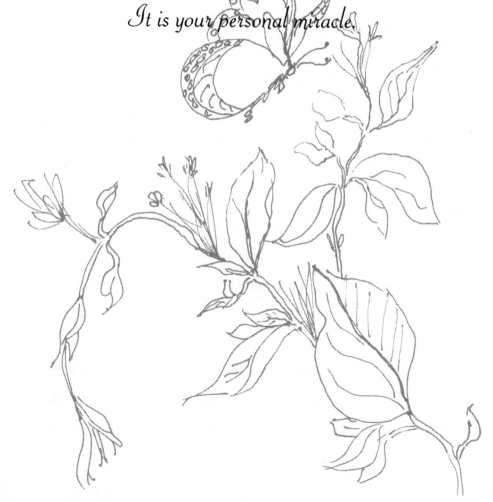

# The Envelope of a New and Eternal You

Your body makes a new layer of skin every few days. Deep in the cells there's a factory constantly working to renew beauty. It's a process that cannot be stopped by fatigue, illness, divorce, or aging. Every week you have a chance to create another you. Each time you clear away an old layer of skin, you eliminate a year of aging.

In your healing space, after your morning laxative tea has worked, stand naked in front of a full-length mirror. Using a soft natural-fiber skin brush, the kind available in health food stores and better pharmacies, brush your skin in long smooth strokes from head to foot. Cover every square inch, including underarms, until your entire body has the same pink glow. Don't be alarmed if your body momentarily gives off an odor. Inflammatory conditions result in that imbalance. As you brush and inflammation is reduced, the odor will clear. It is an important part of the renewal process. Surface fat and deeper microcirculation are being stimulated in order to reduce cellulite. You always release toxins in the process. You will notice results within days. Softer, smoother skin, better circulation, and increased energy will be yours.

# CHAPTER 9

# Let's Get into Shape

*It is no longer enough to be slim: we require more than the fitness of youth.*

*Your Goal:* To lose weight while preventing arthritis, heart disease, and cancer.

*Materials:* A few decorator items and slimming foods for virtual trips. One trip requires white rice, steamed fish, seaweed, Konjac, a Japanese dietary fiber, pots of green tea, Epsom salts, Japanese music and movies, and a skilled massage therapist.

Another virtual trip requires slimming fruits, olive oil, high-intensity sunlamps, Latin music, and sand.

O verweight is a delicate issue. We associate it with aging, poor health, and low sex appeal. Yet no one seems to agree on just how many Americans are overweight. Statistics range from one in three people, to more than half the general population. In the end, it is a matter of personal choice whether or not you choose to lose weight. Would losing pounds make you feel and look better?

Chances are if you lose the weight you have gained from overwork, worry, or chocolate cake, you will feel younger. Your body will remember how you felt before you overdid it. Your mind and spirit will be refreshed.

Do you remember bouncing back from exercise and weight gain like a rubber ball? Getting into shape takes less time and effort when we are young because our metabolism is faster and our recovery time shorter. For that reason, energy-building herbs help you recapture your spark of vitality and allure. Herbs offer many health benefits simultaneously. Certain weight-loss herbs dissolve impurities by enhancing metabolism. This prevents illness because cleansing herbs reduce all sorts of toxins underlying cellulite, arthritis, heart trouble, and tumors.

Thousands of weight loss books have been written. If any of them worked, there would be no more need for such books and no more obese Americans. Obviously the anti-fat industry thrives. Over-the-counter slimming supplements are widely available. Because medical science defines overweight as a disease, the drug industry is busy creating ever more expensive, addictive, and potentially dangerous medicines. Today, while researchers are injecting newly discovered hormones into laboratory mice in order to reduce their appetites, no one knows how human appetites may be affected by such intervention. Is there a connection between hunger for food and hunger for sex or, at least, for social interaction? For us the question remains—If you had a supplement that effectively reduced appetite, would you be any more tempted to eat a healthy diet? You might develop the same diet-related illnesses a bit more slowly.

In China there is no weight loss problem. You can't find weight loss cocktails such as fen-phen—a combination of two prescription drugs, fenfluramine and phentermine, now taken off the market—whose side effects include brain damage, pulmonary hypertension, thyroid problems, and high-blood pressure. Asians are among the longest-lived people on the planet. The average age for Japanese men is seventy-six and, for women, nearly eighty-three. Per capita, more people live to be over one hundred years old in Japan than anywhere else. Considering that, you can't argue with the typical Japanese diet of white rice, sea vegetables, high-fiber foods, shiitake mushrooms, deep ocean fish, and five to ten cups of green tea daily. Now that global communication has shrunk the world, we can benefit from Asia's experience. Japanese products, including concentrated health foods in capsules, as well as Chinese weight loss pills and teas are now available through American distributors listed in the Herbal Access section.

In this chapter we will take several pleasure trips for the purpose of weight loss. Since they are virtual trips, you don't have to leave your home. In addition, beginning on page 166, you can find a comprehensive set of exercises and visualizations that combine Chinese Qi Gong with gentle slimming isometric movements to firm, lift, and reshape you. I suggest herbs to improve your workout results and eliminate pain. Chapter 14 describes a special massage to improve your sexual capacity and the pleasure of being in your body. It will be easy and fun to use all these suggestions together to re-create the one and only original you.

# In Your Healing Space

To start from square one, stand in front of a full-length mirror and observe your body in this special way: cut holes for your eyes in a paper bag and place it over your head. That allows you to look at your body without seeing you. Notice where fat or cellulite has collected.

If fat or cellulite is localized at your waist, hips, and thighs, you may crave sweets, rich foods, or alcohol and have difficult digestion. See the suggestions beginning on page 149.

If overweight is spread through your entire body and you have edema or obesity, you need to adjust your metabolism by stepping up your energy. See the suggestions beginning on page 154.

## A Visualization

Set your mind for your goal: activate your energy to lose weight in this way. Before you begin any diet, take time in your healing space to visualize yourself slim and fit. It may help to look at youthful pictures. Choose a current picture and use a pen to shade areas that need reducing. Keep the slim picture in your healing space as your guide. If the photo is from a happy time in your past, your body and spirit will recall how slender you felt. That will help tone your metabolism.

Imagine yourself at your perfect weight and proportions. Imagine what you would wear while dining on salad in an elegant restaurant. Using a recent photo of yourself, draw an outline within the outline of your body, a thinner shadow body, that you can achieve. Or paste a photo of your head onto another photo of a slim body to get your hormones and enzymes humming. Show yourself the prize.

# Looking Deeper

Take a moment to examine what food means to you emotionally. When do you overindulge? Do you notice a pattern?

I eat or drink more fattening foods

—when I'm tired
—when I'm bored
—when I'm alone
—before my menstrual period
—during cold weather
—all of the above

# Adrenal Weakness and Hunger

People who eat more richly or gain weight when fatigued or during cold weather frequently suffer from adrenal weakness or exhaustion. Before they can have the strength to lose weight, they need to take an energy tonic like the ones I recommend beginning on page 154. Herbal combinations designed to enhance adrenal strength also support vitality and counter exhaustion symptoms, including chronic diarrhea, shortness of breath, pallor, low enthusiasm, and fatigue.

# Emotional Binges and Hunger

People who eat more when they are depressed or bored may need help with their emotions. A number of homeopathic remedies will be beneficial. (See Chapter 16, Heal Your Broken Heart.) For example, for the person who craves sweets, has excess sinus congestion, and often cries over little things, homeopathic pulsatilla 30c is most useful. Add a dozen small white pills to a quart of spring water and drink it throughout the day. It clears up phlegmy congestion and weepy feelings, premenstrual crying, and chocolate binges. It helps balance hormones. Both men and women can use it. Homeopathic pulsatilla improves breathing and energy.

Now that we've established possible causes for your overweight, we need to devise a healing routine to reduce fat and impurities that works specifically for you. Add the recommended homeopathic remedies and herbs for increasing energy as needed to the following programs.

# How to Proceed

• Base your choice of weight loss program on your mirror observation of your body. For fat and cellulite in the midsection, turn to page 149. For obesity or global water retention, turn to page 154.

• Stick with one program for at least a month before you switch to another. You can alternate programs throughout the year in order to protect yourself from a wider range of health and beauty problems.

• Start slowly. Add healthy foods gradually. Do not eat raw or cold foods first thing in the morning, because they weaken digestion. Wait for afternoon to eat raw salads.

• If raw food gives you bloating pain, add one of the digestive remedies I describe on page 151. Also use anti-candida treatments.

• If you have used medical diet drugs that have damaged your heart valve, or if you experience chest pain from cleansing foods or diarrhea, add a capsule of hawthorn to strengthen the heart.

There are many advantages to sane, gradual weight loss. Eventually your addictions will lessen as your body and mind are cleared of impurities. The original you will appear again as out of a seashell.

# A Program of Clearing and Cleansing

Have you ever noticed that both fat and fibroids are lumpy and thick? They have a similar heavy, sticky quality. Plaque that can block blood vessels, causing hypertension, is also a thick, fatty deposit. Arthritis pain is partly caused by wastes like unabsorbed calcium and acids that deteriorate the joints. Many people agree that the conditions underlying asthma, fibroids, and arthritis include inadequate digestion and elimination. A wise diet like the one that follows would reduce fat and normalize weight gain while preventing illness and stress.

# A Simple Wholesome Diet

A basic diet of cooked grains, raw seeds, nuts, soy products (especially tofu), seaweed, salmon, sardines, mackerel, olive oil, digestive fruits such as apple, papaya, and pineapple, as well as vegetables, and natural raw juices normalizes weight gain because it takes digestive stress off the body. The foods are nourishing and cleansing. To this basic diet you can add the recommended raw juices and herbs for special problems based on your mirror observation.

Many low-nutrition foods become addictions because the body can never be satisfied by them. If pasta, pastry, and breads make you puff up with water retention, eat sweet, satisfying, slimming vegetables such as sweet potato and pumpkin. They are grounding and filling but not fattening. You can lose as much as 5 pounds of excess water weight a week by substituting pumpkin pie filling and squash for bread and pasta. Enjoy a breakfast of green tea and spiced pumpkin pie filling. To a 15-ounce can of pumpkin pie filling, add pumpkin pie spice, raw garlic, turmeric, salt substitute, and Sheshecao Instant Beverage used as a sweetener. Enjoy a snack of raw vegetable juice along with air-popped corn with olive oil. Or fast on goat's milk and black figs for a day or more.

# Undo Past Mistakes and Find the Original You

Herbs that rid the body of fat can also help eliminate phlegmy tumors, high cholesterol, and excess acid. Especially useful are bitter cleansing herbs, pungent herbs that increase circulation, astringent ones that dry excess phlegm, and antiseptic herbs that heal infection and clear wastes. If you add generous amounts of the following herbs and nutrients to your diet, metabolism will be increased, and this can help prevent fibroids, arthritis, and heart trouble.

Daily capsules of dandelion, myrrh, hawthorn, and alfalfa as well as edible aloe vera gel added to juice will cleanse the body of acid impurities and strengthen muscles. Barley soup, parsley, celery seeds, squash, and seaweeds such as kombu tone metabolism and reduce congestion. Kava kava, which is actually a pepper, is recommended for depression and obsessive eating. Lecithin, chromium, vitamins $B_6$, C, and E, zinc, folic acid, trace minerals, grape-seed extract, and certain Asian weight loss herbs described in the two weight loss programs that follow are beneficial for reducing cholesterol and normalizing appetite.

To combine weight loss with illness prevention, you need to undo the effects of poor diet and stress with strong cleansing and building foods. Here are a few suggestions for preventing and treating arthritic pain and stiffness. Also see the recipes in Chapter 6 for relief of computer-related pain.

# Lose Weight and Prevent Arthritis

Green vegetables, seaweed, especially kelp and hijiki, and oyster-shell tablets all provide calcium that is much easier to absorb than the calcium in cow's milk. Arthritic pain is directly related to poor digestion and a buildup of undigested impurities in the colon. You can speed and ease digestion greatly by avoiding most dairy products. To remedy pain, add digestive remedies such as bromelain from fresh pineapple or enzyme pills, also laxative herbs such as cascara sagrada and the juices that follow. Also avoid nightshade foods, including tomatoes, eggplant, green bell peppers, garlic, raw spinach (cooked spinach is okay), and white potatoes because they cause a buildup of harmful acid in the joints and muscles. Use cooling spices such as cumin, coriander, and fennel to reduce acid. The best grain for the joints is oatmeal, which is nourishing and cooling. It is especially recommended for rheumatoid arthritis. Add celery seeds.

Supplements useful for arthritic pain include alfalfa, glucosamine, powdered goat whey and herbal combinations such as ArthPlus, made by Nature's Herbs, which contain a variety of anti-arthritis herbs, including devil's claw, yucca, prickly ash, and trace minerals to treat pain and supplement nutrition. Another good combination, called Connect-All, made by Nature's Plus, adds digestive remedies such as bromelain from pineapple and aloe vera to supportive nutritional supplements including vitamin C, zinc, copper, and Chinese sea cucumber to glucosamine and chondroitin sulfate. The latter two ingredients rebuild damaged joints.

During the afternoon and evening, drink a glass of the following raw juice designed to reduce congestion, speed elimination, and treat arthritis pain. To help your digestion, also take a digestive remedy—for example, mint tea.

### Cabbage-Onion Joint Juice

**1 cup aloe vera gel**
**1 teaspoon coriander seed powder**
**1 cup chopped red cabbage**
**¼ cup chopped white onion**
**3 large celery stalks**
**½ teaspoon celery seeds**
**1 handful of fresh parsley**
**1 handful fresh mint or dill**
**1 large cucumber, chopped**
**1 slice raw ginger, 1 inch thick**
**1 tablespoon powdered goat whey**

Place all of the ingredients in a blender and combine until smooth. Add water if necessary. Whey, high in natural sodium, dissolves bone spurs. Mix it with hot water, then blend it with the other ingredients.

Drink a cup of this juice one-half hour before meals. Alternate this with ginger and mint tea or a glass of half cranberry juice, half water. In general, the best way to reduce your appetite is to drink one-half cup aloe vera gel in green tea or juice daily. Aloe is so alkaline and healing and contains such a rich dose of vitamin E that it reduces excess acid—nervous hunger. People with ulcers can add a dash of cumin powder.

If you have arthritis along with high blood pressure and lots of cellulite, drink an additional glass of celery and carrot juice daily. This cabbage-onion juice is similar to my Red-Hot Juice for arthritic pain, carpal tunnel syndrome, and poor circulation in general, but it omits horseradish and ginger, which increase appetite. It adds whey, which is laxative.

# Program One: For Waist, Hips, Thighs, and Sweet Tooth

The following routine includes the basic cleansing diet from page 146 and additional sweet foods that clear the body of mucus and acid. It will improve sluggish digestion and address many health and beauty issues, including arthritis, tumors, asthma, and cellulite.

## How to Proceed

Follow the basic diet, fasting, and slimming wrap suggestions that follow so that your cleansing can proceed uninterrupted during the day. Do not use diuretic herbs and foods at bedtime. This program is designed to reduce your middle bulge fast, so be prepared to adjust dosages to suit your cleansing schedule. The basic diet ensures beauty and longevity and is spartan enough to prevent disease. Here is an important addition that does the trick and is pure fun: I have added several health-building virtual trips to this chapter—one to Miami Beach, another to the California desert, and another to a Japanese health spa. Sometimes a big change in routine is all you need to get started. Getting away for the weekend can be as easy as rearranging your schedule.

# A Virtual Getaway: A Watermelon Fast on the Beach

This is a slimming treat for your sweet tooth. One of my favorite ways to lose puffy water weight is to spend a few days in the Miami heat for a watermelon fast on the beach. You can do it anywhere in a sauna, but I feel reborn on the beach. A watermelon fast is very effective. The fruit is primarily water and minerals, which are laxative and diuretic. You will lose bulges and clear your skin of impurities. Make sure to eat the watermelon seeds and rind—all except for the thin green skin—because they are the most cleansing.

Coconut juice is another healthful fast because of its high mineral content, but I love the taste and texture of watermelon. Because you are eating primarily raw fruit for this fast, you will need to drink two tablespoons daily of raw cold-pressed olive oil or add it to this salad in order to protect your hair and skin from dehydration: slice watermelon, cucumber, and jicama onto a bed of romaine lettuce. Top with olive oil, a dash of lime juice, and powdered chili pepper.

For an at-home Miami trip in your healing space, turn up the heat and add high-intensity sunlamps, aloe plants, and beach pictures. Turn off the phone and play Gloria Estefan records or ocean sounds all day. Spread beach towels on the floor, put on a bikini, and invite some friends over for watermelon. If you prefer being alone, do yoga stretches on your private beach and paint your toenails a nice shade of watermelon.

To imitate Miami's heat, drink enough cinnamon tea throughout the day to make yourself perspire. Prepare it by adding one-quarter teaspoon cinnamon powder to one cup boiling water. Sip it as you eat the watermelon. Rub yourself with a towel so that you perspire from every pore.

Another delicious cleansing and building food is cherries. Big sweet Bing cherries contain large amounts of iron. They are also recommended for gout. Cherry stems are diuretic and recommended to reduce cellulite. Eat a pound of cherries then boil the stems for twenty minutes in one pint of water. Pour the cherry stem water over green tea leaves. This complete fruit—at once a builder and a cleanser—can be an addition to your watermelon fast that reduces fat while it eases pain and stiffness.

## Laxative Herbs

To continue cleansing after your sauna, take the following combination of laxatives. Add one-half cup aloe vera gel to water and take six to eight capsules of dandelion and one capsule of myrrh. If this combination is not strong enough to increase cleansing during the day, add one or two capsules of cascara sagrada, a bitter laxative. Cascara may take up to eight hours to work, but when it does, its flushing action increases peristalsis, the normal spasms of the colon.

## Special Herbs for Bloating and Indigestion

Raw food diets and fasting sometimes cause bloating discomfort. To ease this, digestive remedies that settle the stomach and resolve intestinal gas are helpful. Among these are warming tonic herbs such as ginger used in tea. Otherwise, I like to combine capsules of Shilajit, an East Indian rejuvenation remedy made from processed bitumen, a coal by-product, along with slimming raw fruit or vegetable diets. This heavy, moistening, and carminative mineral attracts impurities from throughout the body to eliminate them. Take two to four capsules daily during a raw fruit fast to flatten your stomach and eliminate gas.

A homeopathic remedy for indigestion is carbo veg. 30c. This vegetable charcoal helps reduce bloating but lacks the Ayurvedic herb's moistening, rejuvenating qualities. In India, Shilajit is recommended for infertility. It renews sexual function weakened from excess dryness. See more information on its sexual benefits on page 192.

## A Slimming Wrap

Some people consider it trendy to have their cellulite wrapped in mud or seaweed. Others have it pounded with massage, smeared with oils, or shocked with electrodes. These efforts are all aimed at dissolving fat deposits by making you sweat. You can do a better job of reducing cellulite in your thighs, waist, and hips at home the following way. (This is best done on an empty stomach and not during your period or while you're pregnant.)

If you don't have a sauna, you can create one in your body that treats specific areas. Spot reduction of fat is possible with localized sweating. If you are very weak or have a health condition that precludes excess sweating, you can still wrap up your cellulite areas while you exercise and drink a cup of cinnamon tea.

1. Saturate your cellulite area with a layer of pure corn oil. Oddly enough, its action is diuretic. (See page 121.)
2. Then wrap the cellulite area—stomach, hips, thighs, or whatever—with three layers of Saran Wrap, like a slimming mummy.
3. Pull on long wool or cotton underwear over the Saran Wrap layer.
4. Then follow this with nylon gym pants, or wrap yourself up in a sheet.
5. Finally, wrap an electric blanket around the area. If you didn't have the layer of Saran Wrap, you'd sweat through the long underwear.
6. To increase sweating, drink a mug of hot cinnamon tea.
7. Soak your feet in a gallon of hot spring water to which you have added the juice of one lemon (organic, if possible).
8. Perspire to your heart's content. Stay in your personal sauna no longer than twenty minutes. Then shower off immediately with warm water. If you feel weakened by losing water weight too rapidly, limit your sauna to ten minutes a day. You will see the benefits in the first week.

You may be wondering how slimming juices and sweating treatments reduce your risk of arthritis, fibroid tumors, and heart trouble. It's simple. Such cleansing increases your metabolism and helps dissolve impurities that can be lodged anywhere in the body. In addition, as we have already seen, you can use these cleansing treatments when you need to detoxify from alcohol, drugs, or chemotherapy.

# Shake and Bake It: A Virtual Trip to the Desert

I know a place where all you can hear is the flow of hot mineral water and birds singing. The sun rises in a blue sky over snowcapped mountains. Yellow, purple, and red flowers grow in sand, and roadrunners streak by as you walk. This desert is far enough from Los Angeles to be out of the freeway—cell phone—name-dropping orbit. You are left in peace with prairie dogs and jackrabbits. The best slimming foods there are sun-drenched fruits—dates, prunes, figs, bananas, and apricots—during the morning and large salads in the afternoon.

I often start the day with dried fruit and a few slices of raw ginger in a pot of green tea, followed by a walk in the desert. Dried fruit that has been soaked to remove excess sugar and hot tea are easier to digest than raw fruit and cold drinks. I may take a capsule of hawthorn to speed diges-tion and brace my energy. I take a long dip in a hot mineral water pool before beginning a day's work at my computer. In the late afternoon I return to the water, a sauna, or the sun. After two weeks of a cleansing diet made up of fresh and dried fruits, vegetables, bean burritos without cheese, and raw tofu fixed with soy sauce and balsamic vinegar, my cel-lulite is noticeably reduced. My bones soak up the sunshine, my favorite source of vitamin D. Other sources include cod liver oil capsules, which I take daily for healthy complexion, vision, teeth, and bones.

After soaking in hot water and letting the whirlpool jets massage my cellulite, I smear Mexican yam cream on my abdomen, inner thighs, and sexual area. This cream, available in health food stores, is a natural source of progesterone—essential for normal hormone balance. Regular use reduces water retention in the lower body and sluggish periods, while it moistens the skin's surface. Remember yam cream in later chapters that deal with sexual satisfaction. It eliminates dryness for women who require lubrication and intensifies sexual response for both partners.

For a virtual trip to the desert, spend the afternoon in a hot mineral water bath. Add Epsom salts to a full tub, scrub briskly with a loofah or washcloth. Enjoy raw pineapple, dried cranberries, prunes, and sunflower seeds while you soak. Later fix a beautiful salad including bitter greens, papaya, mango, cucumber, raw ginger, and lots of celery. Celery reduces cellulite as well as arthritis pain.

## Massage Away Hunger

For anyone stuck for hours at a desk or in an L.A. traffic jam, there are acupuncture points that can reduce nervous hunger. It's easy to massage these points during a bath or while waiting for the next freeway exit. This massage eases muscle tightness affecting the abdomen, thereby reducing hiatal hernia and nervous hunger.

On top of your bare feet are webs formed by the tendons joining the toes to the ankles. Massage inside these webs. The most important points for weight loss are between the webs formed by the first and second toes and the second and third toes. The points will be sensitive. Press firmly one inch above the space between the first and second toe, then one inch above the space between the second and third toe. Then press directly above these, two inches above the space between the toes. In a car, massage the acupuncture points using your hand or the opposite foot. (See the illustration on page 171.) Imagine your stress and hunger flowing downward through the bottoms of your feet.

# Program Two:
# For Obesity and Junk-Food Addictions

If you are generally overweight and can't pass up a cookie or a loaf of bread, you have to proceed more slowly. Extreme fatigue, frequent urination, and low immunity are side effects of being overweight. If that is the case, the earlier programs of fasting and sweating are too extreme for you right now. First, you must build adequate vitality, endurance, and the willpower to lose weight. That, in a nutshell, describes adrenal strength.

This program for weight loss and illness prevention includes teas that reduce harmful cholesterol and protect against heart trouble, energy tonics that increase your sense of well-being, and slimming herbs. While it is designed for people who wish to lose weight, it is suitable for anyone who has chronic illness and poor immune strength. Only after you have gained sufficient strength by following the recommendations in Program Two for at least one month should you consider adding the cleansing fast and wrap of Program One. Otherwise, you may damage your energy and retard weight loss.

# How to Proceed

Barring allergies, follow the basic diet found on page 146 as closely as possible. Although food allergies and yeast infections can be a problem in either Program One or Program Two, I treat it here because it is nearly always associated with chronic fatigue, weakness, and generally poor health.

If you have candida or a yeast or fungus infection with itchy mucus discharges, low energy, painful growling indigestion, and crankiness, temporarily omit foods that encourage yeast: grains, yeast breads, fermented foods, including tofu, and all sugar, including fruit. Eat only vegetables, rice cakes, sprouted bread, fish, almonds, seeds, mineral water, and green tea for three days. You will enjoy this sort of diet when you take your virtual trip to Japan, which I describe later.

This diet alone may not eliminate your yeast problem if it is of long standing or a result of taking antibiotics or birth control pills. In that case, add the following special tea to rid yourself of chronic yeast infections. After the infection is gone, you can go back to the basic diet, adding slimming herbs and teas.

## Anti-Candida Tea

For some people, candida is a lifelong struggle with repeated ineffective doses of expensive Western drugs. Drinking this tea, or using the oil as toothpaste, while limiting your diet of yeast-producing foods can often get rid of candida in three to four days.

**1 drop Australian Tea Tree Oil**
**1 cup hot water**
**1 dose homeopathic belladonna 30c**

It's simple to make and tastes as though it should be used to disinfect the bathroom. The tea tree oil is antifungal, and the homeopathic remedy prevents a headache and fever reaction while the yeast is dying. If you want to make this stronger, take it along with a capsule of goldenseal, another anti-yeast herb that affects the colon, and cascara sagrada, a bitter laxative.

## Important Energy Tonics Just for You

Everyone needs more vitality from time to time, but you may need it more often. In fact, low vitality is at the root of your inability to lose weight. After you have dealt with candida for a few days and are following the basic diet, the following herbal energy tonics will make it easier for you to eat and stay healthy and slim. You will notice that as your energy improves, so will your backaches, depression, asthma, and addictions. You crave fattening foods because your body is weak.

## Vitality Teas

Weak people with edema, pallor, and chills should avoid raw juices until they are strong enough to tolerate them, or else they should drink a small glass in the afternoon along with strong digestive herbs such as cardamom, ginger, and clove.

The following teas are not in themselves slimming, but will increase adrenal strength so that you will feel ready to diet. Add any one of the following herbs to a cup of boiling water to pick up your energy:

—1 teaspoon clove buds or ½ teaspoon clove powder

—1 sprig rosemary herb

—1 sprig fresh garden sage or one teaspoon dried herb

—1 capsule damiana

You will enjoy these bracing teas most at midmorning and midafternoon during what are traditionally the energy low points of the day. Never take these or any warming stimulant herb or food when you have a cold or fever. Use these with caution if you have high blood pressure, palpitations, or menopausal hot flashes.

Here are two additional Chinese favorites you can order from addresses listed at the back of this book. Chinese ginseng, called ren shen or panax ginseng, is a heating stimulant herb that strongly increases the metabolism. If you cook a piece of the dried herb in soups, it warms you and speeds up your metabolism immediately. But you must be careful. You may feel dizzy and hot from this herb if you need an energy tonic that is more cooling and moistening.

Skip Chinese ginseng altogether if you have chronic thirst or hunger, ulcers, and dry skin, and substitute American ginseng tea, called *quinque-folium* in Latin. It is an entirely different plant from Chinese ginseng. Its moistening effects will feel refreshing and satisfying enough to reduce burning hunger. Some people have reported that it reduces sweet cravings. Drink three to five cups daily.

Another Chinese herbal potion widely reputed to help adrenal strength is a patent remedy called Sexoton. Patent remedies are herbal combinations that were patented generations ago. They are safe and quite effective when you know how to use them. This one treats weakness, pallor, shortness of breath, chronic diarrhea, aching lower back, frequent urination, depression, and low vitality. The normal dosage is 6 to 8 small pills three times daily between meals. We will study its ingredients in Chapter 13, Total Energy for Work and Play.

## Slimming Juices

Because your most important weight loss issue right now is maintaining high energy to ensure proper digestion, fresh juices offer you the best kind of stimulation. Ripe citrus fruits have been linked with fibroid prevention because of their vitamin C content. Carrot juice and spinach juice tone liver function to help eliminate water retention.

Used judiciously, these raw juices will give you a rosy outlook and an energy boost, especially during the afternoon. Drinking juiced vegetables first thing in the morning will give you a headache later in the day. Instead, drink the juice between meals in amounts you can easily digest, or try to eat larger meals at breakfast and lunch, saving these juices as a dinner substitute or dessert. Juice the entire fruit but not the skin, which may contain a dye. Though not always available, organic apples are your best choice. Remember to juice fruits *along with the seeds* and *not to mix fruit and vegetable juices during the same day.* Choose one of these meal selections daily. Use only very ripe fruit along with a capsule of lecithin.

—2 grapefruits

—2 oranges

—1 grapefruit, 1 orange, and 1 lemon

—4 carrots, 1 cup spinach

—4 carrots, 1 medium beet, 1 large cucumber, ½ cup parsley

—1 apple, 1 cup lettuce, 1 lemon, ⅛ teaspoon prepared horseradish

# Additional Weight Loss Herbs

Traditional Chinese medicine has devised some handy pill and tea remedies to help you regain your shape. They can be used by anyone and will work better as adrenal strength improves. They can be ordered from sources listed in the Herbal Access section at the back of the book.

Bojenmi Slimming Tea contains hawthorn and other cleansing herbs that tone the system completely. Drink only one cup a day when you start and never more than two. Otherwise the hawthorn may overstimulate your heart to give you a slight headache or the jitters.

I like Obesity-Reducing Tablets (Qingshen Jianfei). Recommended for simple obesity, they are said to strengthen vital energy, enhance the spleen, activate blood circulation, and get rid of any stuffy feeling in the chest. I like them because they are easy to take—four tablets three times daily, and they don't increase my hunger like other weight loss pills. The vegetarian formula contains valuable energy tonic herbs such as astragalus, circulation herbs, including salvia and ligustrum, and cleansing and diuretic herbs.

If you feel you need a diuretic herb to increase urination, make sure that you find one that also contains potassium—for example, Nature's Bounty Water Pill, made by Nature's Bounty in Bohemia, New York. It contains buchu leaves, uva ursi, parsley, juniper, and potassium. Do not take diuretic herbs if you have a lower backache, pale-colored urine, and extreme fatigue. With these symptoms, you still need to build strength with the herbs and foods on page 156.

# A Virtual Trip to Japan

This virtual trip re-creates the order and serenity aimed for in Zen practice. In your healing space find a blank wall and a table. Hang a white or pastel-colored sheet on the wall behind the table. Cover the table with a black or dark-colored cloth. Cut three-foot-long pussy willows or tree branches and put them into an earthenware flowerpot or metal bucket on the covered table. If you prefer, place a large rock or a large glass bowl of water on the table. We want a minimum of lines, colors, and patterns.

The music of a koto, a traditional Japanese string instrument, or a reed flute is particularly soothing. Jasmine or rose incense can help you quiet the space. Watching a slow-paced Kurosawa movie or doing a simple manual activity will help you to relax and enjoy being away from the world. Japanese people have given us wonderful means to good health—sushi, seaweed, Shiatsu massage, and the hot tub. You may want to stay forever.

To the basic healthy diet outlined on page 146, add the following Japanese foods, in capsules, which have been proven effective in lowering fat and cholesterol as they safely reduce hunger.

Take three to six capsules daily of Konjac, made by Pristine and distributed by Intelligent Choice in San Diego. It is best to take one or two capsules along with a whole glass of water or juice before meals. Make sure to take this supplement with lots of water. Called konnjaku in Japan (Konjac mannan), it is a nondigestible fiber that puffs up to forty times its weight in the colon. Frequent use helps keep the colon clean, while reducing cholesterol and hunger. Konjac is not slimy, like psyllium husks and, for that reason, is well tolerated by people with mucus congestion. It makes a good addition to a slimming fast of fruits, vegetables, tofu, and seeds.

Chitosan and Ashitaba are capsules also made by Pristine. The first is made from Japanese zuwai crab shell, a supplement that is enjoying popularity among anticholesterol enthusiasts. It is a fat-soluble fiber used for weight loss and disease prevention. You can combine one or two capsules with Konjac before meals. Ashitaba is a capsule of powdered young angelica *(Angelica archangelica),* which reduces digestive pains, ulcers, and fibroid masses. It is more convenient to take capsules than to brew angelica roots, which taste extremely bitter and smell bad.

As you relax and enjoy the healing process, you will think of other virtual trips to places with simple wholesome diets. You will bask in good weather, exercise, and dance with beautiful people. You may even find the time and freedom to fall in love. The *original you*—the unchanging you— was a sleek, graceful swimmer inside the womb. In previous lives, the energy which is your birthright took shape as a fish, bird, fox, or deer that never worried about calories or cholesterol. Your spirit will remember the spark of energy that began your journey as you clear away the debris made by time.

# Five-Day Plans for Spot Weight Reduction

For spot reduction, focus on these slimming foods: fresh and dried fruits and vegetables, apple cider vinegar, lecithin, chromium, and mixed vitamins and minerals, especially vitamin $B_6$, C, D, and zinc. Do not neglect $B_{15}$ (N-Dimethylglcine, also called DMG), which becomes depleted from increased bowel movements. This nutrient is recommended for enhanced immune response. DMG also improves neural impulses to the brain and is important for certain nerve-related conditions, including migraine headaches and multiple sclerosis. To cleanse and build your blood, drink several glasses of half water and half liquid chlorophyll.

## Abdomen

Choose one of the following teas daily after light meals. The medicinal herbs are individually available from Chinese herb shops listed in the Herbal Access section. You make the combinations.

## *Pinellia Middle-Slimming Tea*

**1 handful of Chinese pinellia buds**
**4 pieces of magnolia bark**
**1 piece of dried orange peel (chen pi), or ½**
    **teaspoon of the prepared spice**
**1 handful of sliced licorice sticks**

Simmer these ingredients for twenty minutes. Drink three cups daily. If this tea gives you cramps, add one handful of sliced raw ginger after boiling and steep the tea at least ten minutes.

Brew a strong green tea and add fresh mint and raw ginger. This tea is tasty and easy to make. Take laxative capsules—two cascara sagrada and three dandelion—with each cup. Drink three cups daily. This will keep you busy cleansing.

Brew Chinese Bojenmi, or The Wellknown Tea, adding one-quarter cup of aloe vera gel per pot. Use laxative herbs or slimming teas containing malva (a laxative), three cups daily or as comfortable. Avoid senna— it causes cramps. People who are diabetic should drink corn-silk tea and eat cooked oatmeal to lower their blood sugars. Pickled nopale cactus served as a side dish will also lower high blood sugar.

## *Middle-slimming foods and activities*

After you've begun using the teas, add lots of middle-slimming laxative foods to your diet, including squashes, pumpkin, greens, pumpkin and sunflower seeds, cooked and raw tofu with soy sauce and vinegar, steamed fish, barley-parsley soup, celery, salad, fennel tea, and grape-seed extract or wine (page 50).

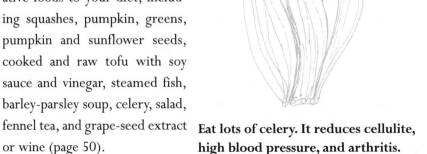

**Eat lots of celery. It reduces cellulite, high blood pressure, and arthritis.**

Exercise! Bend and twist at the middle. Activities such as rowing, tennis, walking, and gym workouts will cause sweating, speed metabolism, and work your muscles.

# Hips and Legs

Drink one of these teas daily between light meals.

> **1 handful of *Stephania tetrandra* (han fung ji)**
> **1 handful of *poria cocos* (fu-ling)**
> **1 pinch of cinnamon powder**

Simmer in one quart of water for twenty minutes. Drink three cups daily. This combination of diuretic herbs especially slims the legs. If you have arthritic knees, add six to ten yucca capsules daily. If you have varicose veins, add two horse chestnut capsules daily. Also see Chapter 6, "Computer-Related Stress and Pain."

Add diuretic and cleansing herbs and foods—cranberry juice and fruit, corn-silk tea, juniper berries, dandelion, alfalfa, parsley, and health food store bodybuilding-slimming combinations that contain healthy stimulant and diuretic herbs. One such product is Razor Cuts, made by National Health Products.

Add stimulant sexual tonics and hormone-balancing herbs in midafternoon—damiana, blessed thistle, and epimedium tea. See Chapter 14 for more information.

## Leg-slimming activities

Exercise: cardiovascular movement such as bicycle and dance reduce bulges. Massage the legs while steaming in a bath or sauna. Pay attention to the inside of the legs, pressing firmly from the groin to the ankles.

## Your ankles and your heart

If your ankles are chronically swollen from water retention, you may have heart weakness. Notice if your energy is low, if you have frequent heart palpitations, shortness of breath, or other symptoms of heart disease. If you have any of these problems, the healthy, slimming anticholesterol diet described previously will be most beneficial. You should also add a heart tonic such as Dan Shen Wan, a combination of Chinese red sage root *(Salvia miltorhizza)* and edible camphor. This pill eases chest pain while increasing general circulation.

---

# Keys

Excess appetite: aloe vera gel in green tea or juice

Sweet cravings: reduce with bitter cleansing herbs—dandelion, aloe vera, gentian extract, skullcap, American ginseng, chickweed

Cholesterol: carrots, celery, garlic, green tea, hawthorn capsules, Chinese slimming teas

**Links:** Also see Chapters 8, 10, 13, 14, 16

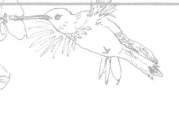

# CHAPTER 10

# Asian Slimming Cures

*To be young is to be fleet of foot.*
*I want ease of movement, grace, endurance,*
*and beautiful muscles.*

---

*Your Goal:* **To reduce bulges, cellulite, and spare tire**
*Materials:* **To cleanse the liver and blood and to rid the body of excess water, use homeopathic natrum sulphate (nat. sulph.) 30c. To eliminate body odors, use homeopathic silicea 30c. Corn oil used during massage reduces fat and increases urination. Wash the oil off after massage.**

---

Most people fixate on losing weight instead of gaining strength. One cannot happen without the other. I have delved into foreign waters, combining several highly effective Eastern energy systems and movements, along with natural products designed to maximize fitness and eliminate pain.

I have begun this chapter with fitness and energy training because poor circulation affects so many Americans. Western medical doctors have come to realize the importance of regular exercise for the prevention of certain cancers, diabetes, and depression. But knowing the statistics never got anyone up from a comfortable chair. It has been estimated that interest in sports during this decade will eclipse money spent on education, travel, and luxuries. The chief editor of *Details* has said that, for young people, sports has become the major American preoccupation, replacing rock music. Whether or not that is true, what about people like me who are not athletic, who would rather attend a play or learn a foreign language than sweat out a refined tennis serve? Is there hope for the athletically challenged?

I found help in an unlikely place. Vermont is not the kind of place where you can easily lose weight. Cooks there specialize in delicious breads, wild-berry muffins, thick pancakes with maple syrup, and gobs of cheddar cheese on just about everything. You can imagine my surprise one summer when I came across a used book on slimming featuring a little-known system of isometric exercise.

The woman author looked fabulous—slim, firm, lifted, tiny bottom, and long, slender legs. Then I looked closer. Her movements required neither complicated machinery nor expensive gym equipment but involved careful movements repeated as many as seventy-five times in a row! I figured she had remained little-known because she had killed her students with exercise. I decided to modify the movements, making them appropriate for cuddly writers who love to eat cookies.

I also stressed isometric exercise involving acupuncture meridians and incorporated traditional Chinese Qi Gong energy balancing. In this way a fitness workout can recondition internal organs and help ensure immunity to illness. *Voilà!* I suddenly thought. Maybe I could even do some of these moves sitting at my computer! Each exercise that is meant for a specific area, such as the waistline or hips, also includes herbal and homeopathic supplements to increase slimming and eliminate workout pain. This program is useful for both men and women, although I have stressed the hips, stomach, and thighs, which are many women's main areas of complaint.

Initiating any exercise program after years of spectator sports can be hazardous, especially if you push yourself too hard in the beginning and then stop. Following my lazy inclinations, I have put together movements, breathing exercises, and herbs that give the most benefit from the least effort. After completing only a day of these movements, you will gain a new sensitivity to your body, especially your posture. You will begin to feel taller, straighter, and stronger.

# In Your Healing Space

Make sure you have lots of sunlight and clean air. Plants increase oxygen during the day. Vines because of their many leaves give off the most oxygen. Why not put an inspiring picture on your altar . . . Tarzan and Jane?

# Ground Rules

Consult your health specialist if you have spinal disk problems or injuries, if you have heart trouble, if you are pregnant, or if you have any other problem that might interfere with exercise.

Make sure to warm up with the stretches and deep breathing described below before you begin the movements. That helps prevent injury and fatigue.

Do not do these muscle-toning movements in a fast, jerking manner.

Establish a time for exercise, and try to be consistent. You don't need to spend more than a couple of hours a week to get great results. Then, when you're satisfied, maintain your shape with fifteen minutes daily.

Exercising in a cold or drafty room causes cramps. If during the movements you get a pain, stop, massage the area and do slow, deep breathing until it stops. Cinnamon tea also helps.

Wait two hours after a meal and one hour after a snack before you begin to exercise.

# Internal and External Warm-Up

The purpose of a warm-up is to stimulate blood circulation in order to increase range and ease of movement. We are going to intensify that experience by using homeopathic remedies that help the body to discharge impurities and receive a full supply of oxygen in the process.

You should use homeopathic potassium, silicea, and iron to increase perspiration and increase oxygen intake throughout the entire exercise period. These minerals are essential for getting enough oxygen into the cells. In turn, oxygen builds energy and fights disease.

Two hours after eating, take one dose each of homeopathic kali. sulph. 6x, silicea 6x, and ferrum phos. 6x, letting them melt under your tongue. Kali. sulph. is potassium sulphate, which clears sticky phlegm. It enhances cleansing by freeing perspiration clogged by mucus. Silicea is the stuff that makes up connective fiber such as hair, skin, and fingernails. It helps clear away toxic debris while it clears the body of odors. Ferrum phos. is the most absorbable form of iron. With the extra oxygen made possible by these remedies, your workout will be more effective and less painful.

You may find it helpful to read the following instructions into a cassette recorder so that you can play them back as you work out.

## Warm-up #1

With your bare feet firmly planted, facing forward, and shoulder width apart, bend your knees slightly to reduce any strain. Stretch up toward the ceiling from your lower back, then your middle back. Place your palms together in front of your chest and stretch your arms over your head, keeping the palms touching. Keep your arms as close to your ears as is comfortable.

Open your palms a few inches, relaxing your fingers. Your hands are like tree branches touching the sky. Your feet are the roots of the tree, gaining nourishment from the soil and sending oxygen to the leaves.

Very slowly inhale from your hands down to your feet, then slowly exhale from your feet up to your hands. Imagine you can watch the breath as it stretches your vertebrae in both directions, making you two inches taller. If you are comfortable, continue breathing in this manner no more than five times, then normalize your breath, letting your arms float to your sides. Stand silently and see yourself as a strong tall tree.

# Warm-up #2

Standing as you did for Warm-up #1, with your knees bent and your feet apart, reach up to the ceiling as you inhale into your lower abdomen. At the top of your reach, inch both arms up two more inches. Put your hands side by side as if you were going to dive into a swimming pool. Inhale and reach for the ceiling; then bend forward, exhale, and reach for the opposite wall until you are bent at the waist.

Release your arms slowly, letting them float down in front of you. Inhaling into your abdomen, hang over from the waist and reach for the floor with your hands. You can bend your knees to reduce the strain. Don't worry if you can't reach the floor.

Inhale and straighten up to a standing position. Take a breath and relax. Then bend your knees and repeat the same stretch upward, outward to the wall, and downward to the floor. Do this exercise five more times. Breathe into your abdomen and rest a moment afterward.

# Warm-up #3

This is a behind-the-knee stretch designed to correct damage done by bad posture and high heels. It realigns sagging internal organs.

Stand barefoot, feet pointing forward, with your toes one inch higher than your heels. This can be done standing halfway on a book or in a doorway with a raised threshold.

Straighten completely without bent knees and in one smooth movement lean forward without breaking in the middle. Stay there breathing slowly to the count of ten. Then return to the upright original position. Do this exercise a total of three times.

# Warm-up #4

Stand firmly rooted with your feet at shoulder width, your knees slightly bent, and your hands over your navel. Inhale by expanding your lower abdomen without moving your chest. Imagine that the exhalation goes down through your legs. Feel the current of air pass through your thighs, knees, ankles, and feet. Do this ten times. If you become dizzy, stop and breathe normally for a moment.

If you are very weak, you can do this warm-up in bed. Place your hands on your navel, inhale gently into the navel, and exhale. Imagine the breath passing downward through your thighs, knees, ankles, and feet. After you've repeated this a few times, stretch out your feet, toes pointing to the ceiling, and relax. Gently turn your ankles in circles to loosen them.

# For the Waist and Stomach

## Digestive Herbs

The natural remedy we will use for the waist is made of two kitchen herbs that increase digestion: ginger and tarragon leaves. It's best to use fresh herbs. Make a cup of tea by steeping a thin slice of raw ginger one inch long and a handful of fresh tarragon. Or use one-quarter teaspoon powdered ginger and one teaspoon dried tarragon per cup hot water. If you have ulcers or acid stomach, substitute one-quarter cup aloe vera gel for the ginger. Drink a cup before you do these exercises.

## Waist and Stomach Movement #1

Stand in an upright position, as you did for the warm-ups, with your knees slightly bent. Put your right arm behind your back as you reach to the ceiling with your left arm. Without bending or twisting your hips, lift upward from your back and left arm and bend at the waist to the right. Reach with your left arm to the right as though you were going to pick something off the wall to your right. Do not straighten up after the stretch but reach one inch farther, then release one inch back. That one inch is your stretch. Repeat the one-inch stretch ten times, without bouncing, then straighten. Repeat the whole stretch five times on each side.

This stretches your waist, abdomen, underarm, and chest muscles. The trick is to increase the number of sets of one-inch stretches, completely relaxing between sets. Work up to ten sets of five one-inch stretches for each side. (For example, 1, 2, 3, 4, 5, breathe, relax. 1, 2, 3, 4, 5, breathe, relax, and so on.)

## Waist and Stomach Movement #2

Stand in a neutral position with feet pointing forward, shoulder width apart. Put your fists on your waist and bend your knees like Yul Brynner in *The King and I*. Without moving your hips, slowly twist to one side as far as you can go, looking behind you. Then twist one more inch, without bouncing. This is easier to do when you lift up at the waist and tighten your buttocks.

Breathing normally, repeat the one-inch stretch five times; then relax and change sides. Work up to ten sets of five stretches and make sure to relax between sets.

## Waist and Stomach Movement #3

Lying flat on the floor or in bed, bend your knees and place your feet flat, pointing forward in front of you. Make sure to touch your lower back to the floor during the entire exercise. Take a few deep relaxed breaths into your abdomen.

Without any jerking movements, lift off the floor, as one unit, your head, neck, shoulders, and chest. Keep them still as if they were all one piece. Now bend forward toward your knees from under your breast, only one inch. This moves the shoulders only slightly toward your knees. That is your stretch. It does not harm the neck but tones the entire abdominal area from the chest to the pubic bone. With this stretch you will be strengthening deep abdominal muscles that you don't normally use.

Repeat this only ten times the first day. Make sure to relax completely. On the following days do five sets of ten stretches, each followed by a count of ten to relax.

The relaxation between exercise sets allows the muscles to respond by strengthening. The abdomen is crisscrossed by a number of muscle groups that are toned from the top down. As you tone one set of abdominal muscles, another set will become engaged and feel sore. Your exercise discomfort will gradually move downward as you tone new muscle groups. There is no need to strain and do wrenching sit-ups. These one-inch stretches will tone your abdomen in one month or less.

# Massage Follow-Up

After each set of stomach stretches, massage the acupuncture points in both your feet in order to reduce water retention and appetite.

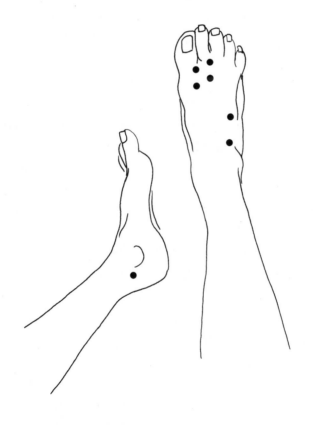

---

## ❧ Herbal Pain Relief ❧

To eliminate muscle pain from exercise or injury, I recommend a Chinese patent remedy used to heal wounds, bruises, and painful swelling called Yunnan Paiyao. It is available by mail order from

Chinese herbal sources listed at the back of this book. Keep it on hand for serious injuries and read about its uses after surgery on page 94.

# Thighs and Legs

## Herbs for Healthy Intestinal Bacteria

The herbs we are going to use for the legs and thighs strongly increase circulation and balance the internal environment of the colon.

Add one-quarter teaspoon of turmeric powder to a cup of warm water and drink it before you exercise. Turmeric is used in East Indian cooking as a digestive spice and for its attractive yellow color (it will stain your clothes and tongue). It's a natural antibiotic that rebuilds healthy intestinal bacteria damaged from illness and antibiotics. You will also feel how effectively it increases circulation in your legs. One-quarter teaspoon taken in water or green tea after meals three times daily can remove even stubborn bruises in less than one week.

My second suggestion may seem strange or at least unorthodox. It is optional. The colon and thighs are related. The muscles in the thighs directly reflect the health of the acid-alkaline balance of the colon. If the colon is ineffective in absorption, then the result is lots of cellulite and poor muscle tone. Increasing intestinal bacteria will help absorption. One of the best ways to increase healthy intestinal bacteria is to take capsules of acidophilus, a health food store digestive remedy. The best way to absorb acidophilus is directly from the colon in an enema or by using a capsule as a suppository. Moisten one capsule of acidophilus with a bit of aloe vera gel and insert it. It won't fall out. This can be done before bed if that's convenient. Important note: If you suffer from chronic joint pains, digestive cramps, skin rashes, or other problems frequently associated with milk allergies, use non-lactose acidophilus. When your body is not struggling with an allergy you have more energy for digestion and circulation. That improves your chances of reducing cellulite.

After following these recommendations, adjust your diet to add more vegetables (especially celery), tofu, fish, seeds, and lots of green tea. Eliminate red meat, cow dairy products, fried foods, and unessential fats and sweets. Also practice the exercises that follow. You will greatly reduce your cellulite, if not eliminate it completely, in six to eight weeks.

# Movements

These movements, breathing exercises, and visualizations originate from Qi Gong, a traditional Chinese system of healing that strengthens vital energy within internal organs and their pathways. Qi Gong styles vary, but they all use subtle movements directed at sending vitality inward instead of building muscles. To a basic Qi Gong movement that aims to build sexual strength, I've added a small isometric movement that will shape your legs, firm your buttocks, and free rejuvenating hormones.

## Thigh and Leg Movement #1

The movements for thighs and legs can be done at a barre or sturdy table-top. Eventually you can do these movements without support.

Clasp the back of a chair or kitchen counter with both hands, shoulder width apart. Put your heels together, with your feet and legs pointing out to either side. It looks like a relaxed ballet first position with a comfortable bend in the knees. Stand on the balls of your feet, keeping your heels together if you can. Lift your head and straighten your back.

Find your balance, release your grasp, and open your hands, allowing the edge of your hands to remain on the chair for support. You will look as if you're holding a large beach ball while standing with bent knees and on the balls of your feet with your heels close.

Tighten your buttocks and inhale as though through your hands. Direct the breath down to your pelvis. As you receive the breath, tilt your pelvis up as high as you can. Hold the breath in your tilted pelvis for a second, then send that energy up to your third eye (located between your eyes). Release your pelvis, returning it to the straight starting position as you exhale.

Repeat this five times; then lower yourself one inch by bending your knees. You may have to separate your heels as you bend lower. Repeat the inhalation and tilt, sending energy to your third eye, and straightening as you exhale in one long continuous breath, lowering yourself one inch after each set of five. Do three sets of five inhalation-tilt-exhalations while lowering yourself, followed by three more while rising up to your original position on the barre. You will really feel it in your thighs. Your shoulders should remain level and your back straight throughout the movements.

## Thigh and Leg Movement #2

This is a simpler version of the one above. Facing the barre or the back of your chair, hold on with both hands at shoulder width apart. Rise up onto the balls of your feet, knees and feet pointing outward, heels together. Keep your back as straight as possible. Holding your head high, lower your body three inches and no more. Do not drop your heels. Keep your body straight. Go back to your original position and repeat for a total of ten times.

## Massage Follow-Up

Your thighs and buttocks will ache after these movements, so give them a warming massage with a few drops of oil. The best oils for slimming are corn or safflower. Also massage around, on top of, and in back of the knees. Rub hard three inches above the kneecap in front. There are acupuncture points above and on both sides of the knee, which increase circulation. Massage the thighs in long upward movements, then loosen the calves, ankles, and feet with massage. Soak your feet in hot water to which you have added one-eighth cup grated raw ginger or one tablespoon dried ginger powder. (Also see the anti-cellulite home sauna on page 151.) Follow this by rubbing your knees and ankles with ice. Pat dry.

# Inner Thighs

This is a modified version of a traditional Chinese movement recommended to tone the muscles after childbirth. We will add a pelvic tilt and special breathing to use it for the inner thigh. This exercise can be done standing or lying flat. Be gentle when you start, to avoid stressing your back.

## Inner Thigh Movement

Stand with your feet apart at shoulder width and your knees bent. Point your feet inward toward each other as far as you can, with your bent knees and big toes a few inches apart. You can feel a stretch behind your legs. Lift your big toes off the floor and point them up toward you for a count of ten.

Keeping your knees bent and legs turned inward, straighten your back and take a breath into the lower abdomen. It may help to look into a mirror for balance.

Inhale into your lower abdomen, and as you exhale, tilt your pelvis up, tightening your buttocks. Don't stick your behind out when you exhale. Drop the pelvis straight as you inhale through your nose; tilt it up as you exhale through your mouth. You may want to puff the air out with a sound.

Do this stretch and tilt slowly for ten repetitions; then relax in place for a count of ten, and begin again. The first day do a total of fifteen repetitions. Then, as it is comfortable, increase them up to no more than thirty. The most important thing is not the number of repetitions but the stretch and breath as well as your mental concentration during the movement. Imagine that your inner thighs and sexual area are being lifted through the top of your head. Then relax completely.

## Massage Follow-Up

End all your exercise sessions with a brisk foot massage and hot bath. If you feel dizzy from newly freed circulation, sit and breathe deeply for a moment. One dose of homeopathic nat. sulph. 30c (natrum sulphate) under the tongue, or ten drops of the bitter cleansing herb skullcap added to a little water will help clear your head because they cleanse the liver of impurities released during exercise.

The exercise that my rejuvenation workshop participants have enjoyed the most is the one on page 173. It takes a little practice to find your balance and coordinate the breathing. When you do, it becomes a smooth, thrusting movement.

Using primarily that movement during a semi-fast, eating only the slimming foods mentioned in Chapter 9, I lost nearly ten pounds in two weeks. It felt great.

# Keys

Pain and injury: Yunnan Paiyao, homeopathic arnica 30c
Gym odor: Homeopathic silicea
Massage oils:
    Slimming—corn oil
    Cooling—sunflower or safflower
    Relaxing or grounding—sesame, olive
    Antidepression—pure essential lavender oil

**Links:** Also see Chapters 5, 8 (spring and summer), 9, 13, 14

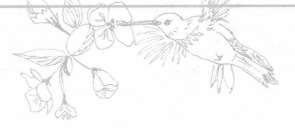

# CHAPTER 11

# Defy the Law of Gravity

*The water inside you is an ocean.*

*Your Goal:* **To reduce wrinkles and improve circulation.**
*Materials:* **Pure essential sandalwood oil, Chinese red jujube dates, astragalus, dang shen, and homeopathic silver (argentum nit. 6x). Optional: herbs to cleanse blemishes.**

Floating completely alone in a swimming pool one long afternoon while facing the sun, I lost track of myself and became part of the water. Weightless, shapeless, my internal organs floated like bubbles. I felt free of gravity's downward pull. We struggle against its force unaware: growing upward in youth, we age sagging downward. For the afternoon, I was released from the bonds of time.

The freedom I experienced while floating in that pool is the feeling of perfect circulation, the sort of relaxation that would be possible if blood and energy were allowed to flow uninterrupted, reaching all areas of the body by means of its normal pathways. In this chapter we will learn to accomplish this with herbs. We can reverse gravity's pull by applying acupuncture principles. Acupuncture aims to redirect and facilitate circulation in order to heal the body. Herbs also affect energy pathways, lifting what has fallen with time and wear.

A sort of energy balancing can be accomplished with certain oils and massage techniques that move circulation. We all have experienced the pleasure of being stroked in a particular direction, for example, downward from the head, over the shoulders, and toward the lower back. We find it soothing because it lengthens tense back muscles. For the face- and body-lifts in this chapter, we will stimulate circulation in the opposite direction to ensure more revitalizing blood flow to the head.

Many people try to reverse wrinkles with surgical or chemical face-lifts. The advantage in using natural means is that herbs can protect the heart and all aspects of circulation. Herbal lifts neither interfere with normal circulation nor leave scars. Herbs cost less than surgery and can be used at home. You may wish to repeat the following energy face-lift anytime you feel low.

# In Your Healing Space

We are going to lift blood circulation and wrinkles using acupuncture meridians without applying needles, lasers, or any medical device. The method I describe is not appropriate for people who frequently feel dizzy, nauseated, light-headed, extremely weak, or enraged. It might feel uncomfortable for anyone with a headache or high blood pressure.

While lying in a hot bath or on your bed, breathe deeply and slowly into your lower abdomen for ten minutes, while gently massaging your abdomen in clockwise strokes. If you are in a bath, add ten drops of pure essential lavender oil to the water. If you're lying in bed, place a few drops of the oil on your abdomen as you massage. Let the spicy lavender scent penetrate your senses.

Take a moment to send any sick, angry, or evil influences in your life out through your feet and down the drain or through the floor. Say goodbye to the problems and people who are troubling you. When you feel clear and calm, continue breathing deeply until you relax completely.

## Sandalwood Oil Cools and Lifts Energy

Place a drop of pure essential sandalwood oil on the very top of your head. This was the neonatal font, the soft spot in the middle of your scalp that was the last part of the skull to fuse after birth. Sandalwood, a cooling oil that attracts circulation to itself, lifts your energy to that spot. It activates a deep acupuncture meridian, which passes through the uterus or testes, abdomen, stomach, heart, and brain, lifting its energy toward your neonatal font. You may feel temporarily flushed after placing the drop of oil on your head. Relax and allow your energy to move freely.

As this is happening, focus on a loving thought, a prayer, or a healing image. Allow your spirit to leave through the top of your head and merge with your favorite deity or highest inspiration. Keep that image on top of your head as you continue to breathe.

# Herbs to Protect Circulation and the Heart

No one associates the heart with beauty. Most people consider a clear complexion, luxuriant hair, a lithe body, or a sparkling personality to be worthy of admiration, while they consider the heart merely an engine that keeps the beautiful chassis running. Without a strong heart, however, oxygen cannot nourish the complexion, youth fades, facial luster dulls, and the mind and emotions go limp.

One way to ensure adequate circulation is to supplement important vitamins, including C, E, and beta carotene, rutin, and also minerals such as calcium, iron, and trace minerals. Drinking green tea instead of coffee helps strengthen blood vessels and protects their elasticity. But there are other things you can do to protect your heart and to preserve the glow of youth.

The following heart tonic herbs protect you from stress, hardening of arteries, fatigue, and chest pain. They are an excellent tonic for older persons with a weak heart and water retention in the midsection. And they are safe for people with hypertension and poor circulation. Using these tonic herbs daily can promote beauty, longevity, and emotional balance.

## Susan Lin's Heart Tonic

Susan and Frank Lin, owners of Lin Sisters Herb Shop in New York City's Chinatown, have been my closest Chinese-American friends for many years. I've sent hundreds of people to them for expert herbal advice and acupuncture. This is one of Susan's herbal concoctions made from major Chinese tonic herbs. It is a health food to protect heart vitality that I recommend for fatigue, large waistline, and high cholesterol. You can buy it powdered at their shop at 4 Bowery or duplicate it in Chinatown herb shops anywhere in the world. Add one teaspoon of the powder to juice daily.

The powder is made from equal parts of salvia, white peony, raw tienchi ginseng, safflower, schizandra, astragalus, and ligusticum, along with one piece of high-quality Chinese ginseng. You could boil all the ingredients together for forty-five minutes and drink two cups a day, but buying the prepared powder saves a lot of trouble and money.

In this formula the herbs that increase blood circulation are salvia, tienchi, safflower, peony, and ligusticum. The ones that build strength and resistance are Chinese ginseng and astragalus. Astragalus, mildly diuretic, reduces water retention, while schizandra prevents excess sweating from weakness. Together they fortify your body, helping it "hold in" vitality.

# An Herbal Face-Lift

Some years ago I learned about a delicious easy-to-make wrinkle cure from a lady acupuncturist in Hong Kong. Since then Hong Kong has changed hands, I've lost touch with my doctor friend, and haven't followed her advice concerning her wrinkle tonic. The one time I did try it, it worked wonders, lending the freshness of improved circulation to my skin, leaving my face younger, brighter, and slightly flushed.

I think I'll try her facial toning herbs again this autumn, after a summer of cleansing impurities. The herbs are diaphoretic, so they increase sweating. I wouldn't want to stimulate sweating until I had cleansed impurities and excess acids because diaphoretic herbs send blemishes to the surface of the skin. Before you try the following herbal face-lift, cleanse your skin from the inside out, using my suggested herbal blemish cleanser for a week or two.

# Stage One: Cleanse Blemishes

Start by clearing blemishes—simplify your diet for a week or more. The basic diet on page 54 includes low-fat, non-congesting foods and no caffeine or alcohol. If you need a laxative, take one-half cup aloe vera gel in apple juice or green tea daily, adding one teaspoon turmeric powder. Turmeric is a useful antibiotic that rebuilds healthy internal digestive energy. Also take 50 mg zinc daily to reduce acne.

Other useful blemish-cleansing herbs you may want to use at this time include dandelion capsules taken along with honeysuckle flower tea, burdock capsules, gotu kola capsules for nervous outbreaks, or a skin-cleansing combination of herbs such as Lien Chiao Pai Tu Pien, available by mail order from Chinese herb shops.

After you are satisfied with your cleansing routine, you can begin lifting your wrinkles and toning your face with three Chinese tonic herbs. As you'll see, they can be prepared either as a tea or as a medicinal liquor.

# Stage Two: Energy Lifts

*Astragalus, dang shen, and jujube red date*

The Hong Kong doctor's original face-lift recipe included astragalus, an energy tonic that lifts vitality and normalizes sweating, and dried jujube, a large Chinese red date that tones the heart, building energy. Together astragalus and jujube take increased blood circulation to the skin. I have added an additional herb, Chinese false ginseng (dang shen) to make sure the lifting effects act more strongly on the face. You should avoid this formula when you have a fever, headache, dizziness, or a cold; at those times you should use anti-inflammatory herbs instead.

# Face-Lift Tea

If you decide to use the three herbs as a decoction, you will have to simmer them for at least forty-five minutes. Use one handful of each herb per one quart spring water in a ceramic-coated, glass, or stainless-steel pot. *Avoid aluminum and Teflon.* Drink the resulting brew hot or cold between meals; these herbs can cause digestive stress when taken too close to meals. The combination of astragalus, dang shen, and jujube may make you perspire. It will certainly send your energy to your skin, not to your digestive organs.

## Face-Lift Wine

This is a delicious way to look and feel better. It can become addictive. The preparation of this sweet liquor takes two weeks. You should start it aging while taking your blemish-cleansing herbs.

Cut one handful of astragalus into half-inch pieces with scissors. The dates can remain whole. Add them all to one quart of vodka or dry vermouth in an airtight glass bottle. Keep this away from light and heat for two weeks. Once a day, gently turn the bottle upside down to mix the ingredients with the liquor. By the end of two weeks the liquor will have turned gold and will have a sweet aroma and taste.

The normal dosage for this beverage is one small wineglass daily between meals. Diaphoretic herbs slow digestion if taken with meals. This warming and relaxing drink would also make a lovely gift to share with friends. If you wish to sweeten it further, add a little raw honey. With the money that you save on a surgical face-lift you can visit Asia. If you still decide that you want to go under the knife, see Chapter 7 for herbs you can take to speed healing.

## A Great Body-Lift in a Pill

My unique contribution to alternative medicine seems to be my highly unorthodox combinations of traditional Asian medical potions with health foods to make highly effective beauty remedies. Here is one of my famous recipes. It combines energy- and immunity-boosting herbal tonics, royal jelly, moistening herbs, and homeopathic remedies. It tones and lifts energy, circulation, and immunity as though the sack containing your internal organs and skin were tightened and lifted. If you have become run-down enough to feel your tailbone stab when you sit down or to feel your face and vitality droop from fatigue, if you have lost your youthful sparkle, this is your best formula for renewal. If you have been ill, you may have to use it for three months before you can see and feel the results.

For the moment, the following body-lift formula is a combination of pills and make-it-yourself herbal tea, but I'm always creating new combinations.

# AstroLift

This formula gets its name from one of its principle ingredients: astragalus, a Latin word for a Chinese variety of vetch normally used to build immune strength. The formula is made by combining astragalus, ligustrum, ganoderma, Siberian ginseng, codonopsis, schizandra, licorice, oryza, Chinese malt, and a tea made from simmering American ginseng and ophiopogonis. Then you take a dose each of fresh royal jelly, a highly concentrated form of B vitamins, and homeopathic argentum nit. 6x for younger skin, all together three times daily between meals.

Here's how to make it simpler: the first nine ingredients come in a pill called Astra 8, made and distributed by Health Concerns in Oakland, California. The dosage is five pills three times daily. Make a tea by simmering one handful each of American ginseng and ophiopogonis, both moistening herbs, in one quart of spring water for fifteen minutes. Take five Astra 8 pills with one cup of this tea between meals.

Then you might eat one level tablespoon of raw royal jelly—the real stuff, a bitter paste, excellent though a bit expensive—or you can swallow a vial of the royal jelly sold in Chinese food and herb shops. Finally, take a dose of homeopathic silver, argentum nit. 6x, which is moistening and rejuvenating. Any one of these ingredients will improve vitality and looks, but the combination brings energy, moisture, and freshness to the skin, tones internal organs, and lifts everything that sags.

If you don't have time for all that because you're too busy doing the slimming exercises in Chapter 10 or taking special baths to renew your skin (page 72), here's an even simpler regime: take a handful of Astra 8 pills along with a dose of homeopathic argentum nit. 6x between meals three times a day. Or you can make a decoction by simmering one handful each of astragalus and jujube in a quart of water for twenty minutes. Drink a cup of that, adding the homeopathic silver. You can store the astragalus-jujube tea in the refrigerator for a few days. With your renewed glow of youth, you'll have better things to do than make tea and take pills.

---

# Keys

*First:* Cleanse skin with honeysuckle and dandelion tea, one to three cups daily for several days or as needed.

*Second:* Lift face with astragalus, dang shen, and jujube tea or astragalus-jujube wine.

Lift vitality and immunity with AstroLift tea. The simpler form contains Astra 8 pills, American ginseng, royal jelly, and homeopathic argentum nit. 6x.

**Links:** Also see Chapters 4, 6, 8 (autumn and winter), 13, 14 (massage)

# CHAPTER 12

# No Fear of Fifty

*Dancing flamenco is like having glorious sex in painful shoes. I shall grow old stamping my feet and tossing my head: I shall run away with the Gypsies.*

*Your Goal:* **To find new ways to increase beauty, vitality, and sensuality after age fifty.**

*Materials:* **American ginseng tea, *Polygonum multif.* (he shou wu) pills or liquid extract, and wild yam cream for moisture. Herbs and foods that increase natural estrogen and testosterone for beauty and resilience.**

As you seek mature beauty and health, you will find new doorways to youth. This chapter is intended for anyone interested in a natural approach to hormone balance, which suits current lifestyles. For women, I cover typical menopausal complaints such as hot flashes, irritability, and fragile bones in a way that will help determine which remedies, among the traditional Chinese patent remedies and modern health food store alternatives, are best. For men, I have included natural sources of male hormones for improved energy and vitality.

Energy and sexuality are not, strictly speaking, menopausal issues, but they are strongly influenced by hormonal and emotional changes. Prompted by huge hormonal shifts, menopause can be a time of emotional fire and ice.

My own perimenopausal roller coaster—the year or so before menstruation stopped—was charged with decisions concerning sexuality. My mother had given birth to my brother while on the brink of menopause. Pressed by my own desire for completion, I took my frustrating love entanglement by the horns and threw it out the window. Once I began living as a single woman for the first time in years, my hormones soared— my breasts grew larger, and my complexion glowed—while I took estrogenic herbs including black cohosh. It was as though I learned about my body all over again. I have maintained that hormonal plenty with rejuvenation secrets I will share with you.

When I finally returned to the love of my life, it was with renewed passion. Having passed through the fires of rejection, blame, and forgiveness, our love became closer and deeper. We rediscovered our undeniable, life-giving sexual and spiritual union. With his help, I decided to write a book instead of having a baby. I hope that you find as much happiness as I did in becoming young again.

Not all menopausal stories end so well. I once met a fiery woman who bragged that her menopausal hot flashes were power surges. She believed so strongly that she could affect menopause with her mind that she formed a neighborhood women's support group to instruct members how to overcome hot flashes with a change of attitude. While I admire her spunk, I can tell you that's not enough. Inflammation and blood deficiency, with signs including hot flashes, fever, thirst, and night sweats should be addressed with diet, herbs, and sometimes acupuncture. Otherwise, the heat can boil over. Given stress and weakness, temporary hormonal changes can become chronic problems. We have to learn how to cool down. The lady with the discussion group did not know how to use herbs to cool her menopausal heat wave. Unfortunately, I heard she had a stroke.

# Menopause and Your Energy

Asian herbal doctors consider menopausal discomforts to be feverish symptoms resulting from weakness and hormonal imbalance. Herbs that are available anywhere in the world, when you know how to use them, can reduce internal heat, or underlying inflammation. Many women born in the West passively expect to get menopausal symptoms because they do not realize the relationship between their inflammatory discomforts and their lifestyle. You do not have to suffer hot flashes, night sweats, irritability, and vaginal dryness during perimenopause or after menopause. You can also protect your heart and joints with herbal medicines.

The basic difference between an Eastern and Western approach to menopause is in how symptoms are explained, observed, and treated. In China, foods and herbs that eliminate underlying imbalances are used in place of synthetic hormones, because that approach is safer and costs less. Menopause is a normal healthy process, but unwise life choices cause physical and emotional pain during that time. Here are some basic guidelines to prevention of menopausal discomfort.

# Put Out the Fire

The heater is inside you. Whenever you have hot flashes, fever, insomnia, irritability, and nervousness after menopause (or at any other time during your life), it is because your body has become too acidic. This is equally true for men and women. Excess acid or inflammation can also occur after exercise, smoking, or drinking and as a result of jet lag.

Ways to cool down immediately include the following:

—Stop eating hot spices and garlic.

—Give up caffeine, especially coffee and black tea.

—Stop smoking.

—Stop or reduce drinking alcohol except for an occasional glass of red wine.

—Eat lots of green and yellow vegetables.

—Find sources of natural estrogen and calcium (pages 193 and 195).

—Take twenty drops of skullcap extract or two skullcap capsules three times daily. This herb reduces liver inflammation.

If you change your habits, you are less likely to develop hot flashes, and you will lessen your chances of getting inflammatory arthritis. If you drink five to ten cups of green tea or a noncaffeine tea daily and follow a wise low-fat diet, you will reduce your chances of developing heart trouble and fibroids. If, after making these changes, you still have menopausal symptoms, you need to use herbs to cool the internal heat. I explain a number of cooling and moistening herbal combinations beginning on page 190.

# Using Herbs and Foods That Are Right for You

There are excellent herbal products on the market that eliminate menopausal complaints while providing vitality, sexual strength and endurance, and longevity. Herbal remedies are like foods. Often plants are nourishing and moisturizing as well as stimulating. When using an herbal rejuvenator, the trick is to choose the right herbs for you: everything is in the diagnosis. No two people are alike. Single-herb remedies are often powerful enough to be felt after one or two doses. If you make a mistake you will feel it right away, and it won't leave lasting traces. Here are some general guidelines to help you determine the right herbs for you.

Herbs are described as either warming or cooling because they affect body temperature and metabolism. In general, warming herbs should not be used during fever or for chronic inflammatory conditions. If you have the flu, irritability, insomnia, or hot flashes, using Chinese ginseng (panax), may give you a temporary headache or fever because it speeds up the metabolism, increases energy, and is considered warming. If you have a cold or the flu, using Chinese ginseng can make you feel worse by increasing inflammation. Here are more pointers to help you find the right herbs to restore your youth.

# Is Your Energy Hot and Dry or Cold and Weak?

Traditional Asian medicine has many methods of observation and diagnosis. Some are simple enough to be everyday tools. One method we used in Chapter 3 was facial diagnosis. Another method is on page 204. For now, as a simple experiment, try this Asian tongue diagnosis.

Observe the color of your tongue, using indirect sunlight before brushing your teeth in the morning or at least one hour after eating a meal. You need to notice the color of your tongue when it is not stained by the dyes used in some foods and drinks. The color of your tongue indicates the state of your metabolism, and it will not vary much from day to day.

## Dry Red Tongue

If your tongue looks dry and red, it indicates inflammation and dehydration. Your metabolism tends to be fast. You may have a temporary fever condition or dehydration from hot food or weather. The color of the tongue is a good indicator of general health because it changes according to your diet and habits. When you have a dry red tongue, you need cooling, moistening herbs and foods—for example, he shou wu, or American ginseng (*quinquefolium*)—to increase your body fluids. Hopefully, after a while, you will have a normal pink tongue, not a dry red one. More important, your underlying condition will have changed so that you will be less likely to have hot flashes, irritability, insomnia, ulcers, and headaches.

## Pale, Puffy Tongue

A pale tongue indicates weakness and slow metabolism. The tongue may also be large and puffy or have ridges at the sides left by your teeth. This kind of tongue is waterlogged from slow digestion, chronic heart weakness, or fatigue. If that is the case, warming tonic herbs such as Chinese ginseng or East Indian ashwagandha are the best way to ensure vitality.

Using tonics—herbs that rejuvenate weak or damaged organs—instead of stimulants such as caffeine, is wise, because tonics do not wear out the body by overstimulation. After using warming tonic herbs for a while you will notice that your tongue returns to a more normal pink. You will be less likely to develop depression, shortness of breath, fatigue, and aches and pains that feel worse in cold, damp weather.

Choosing the right herb or herbal combination can be as simple as that. One of the rewards of using this extremely simple self-diagnosis is that you get to know your energy so you can choose the best possible foods and medicines. In the following section, I have described a number of popular Asian and Western herbal remedies. Using your observations and self-knowledge, you can determine which are useful for you.

# Cooling, Moisturizing Herbs for Men and Women

The following herbal products can be used by either sex because they do not affect hormonal balance. Anti-inflammatory products useful for flushed appearance, chronic thirst, tight lower back muscles, red, dry tongue, hot flashes, night sweats, and sexual dryness include moistening, blood-building herbal combinations. I have provided vegetarian Chinese and Ayurvedic pill remedies. By choosing one of these nourishing herbal pills you ensure vitality, radiant skin and hair, renewed sexual fluids for vaginal comfort, and increased semen.

You may want to call in your order, or photocopy this page and fax it to your favorite Asian herb shop or one that I have listed at the back of the book. (For my friends who enjoy languages, I've provided an Herbal Pronunciation Guide beginning on page 290.)

Liu Wei Di Huang Wan (Six Flavor Tea) is an ancient Chinese formula, originally recommended for hypertension and diabetes, made up of roughly equal amounts of raw rehmannia, cornus fruit, dioscoria root, moutan bark, poria, and alisma. You might buy an ounce of each of these dry herbs and simmer a handful of each in a quart of spring water for forty-five minutes, but it's easier to swallow a handful of the tiny bitter-sweet pills three times daily.

This nourishing blood-building formula has been used by both sexes for many generations to reduce weakness and pain in the lower back, insomnia, afternoon fevers, sensations of burning heat in the soles or palms, night sweats, dizziness, tinnitus (ringing in the ears), chronic thirst, sexual dryness or blood deficiency–related impotence or low sexual response, high blood pressure, and certain problems associated with diabetes.

Liu Wei Di Huang Wan is an excellent all-around tonic for persons who are overheated and dry. Its moistening effects prevent burnout. Normal dosage is eight to fifteen pills or more three times daily. Stop taking this or any moistening or blood-building herbal formula when you have a cold or flu. You don't need to increase moisture, which could lead to sinus congestion.

Zhi Bai Ba Wei Wan (Eight Flavor Tea or Anemarrhena, Philodendron, Eight Flavor Pill) is a variant of the above Six Flavor Tea, containing two additional liver-cleansing, anti-inflammatory herbs, philodendron bark and anemarrhena rhizome. Philodendron is used for inflammation of the lower body with burning yellowish discharges, while anemarrhena is recommended for inflammation in the upper or entire body such as fever.

If you are susceptible to irritating yeast infections, yellow or burning discharge, or sexual discomfort from dryness, you can take three or four handfuls of these small pills daily until the symptoms subside.

Quiet Contemplative-Kidney Yin is also based on Liu Wei Di Huang Wan, but it's made in America by Jade Pharmacy. Like the classic Chinese formula, it treats problems associated with being overheated, including dry skin or mouth, dry eyes, night sweats, and hot flashes.

It contains additional herbs such as lycium fruit, he shou wu, and eclipta leaf to recondition a stressed liver. Eclipta is a fine tonic for people with damaged bone marrow, cirrhotic livers, and hair loss resulting from illness or chemotherapy.

The recommended dosage is two to six tablets daily or ten to twenty drops of liquid extract in a little water taken between meals.

# Shou Wu Pien

On page 226 I describe various forms of he shou wu *(Polygonum multi-flori),* a very useful herb for reducing thirst, mouth dryness, skin irritation, and premature gray hair associated with moisture and blood deficiency. The pill form is called Shou Wu Pien. It is a major herb indicated for menopause or dryness in either sex. Use it wisely and it will replenish youth and beauty. Overuse can cause excess mucus, slow digestion, and water retention. The average dosage is five pills three times daily, but there is no "average" person. You have individual needs. The best way to know how many moistening pills to take is to observe yourself. The best dosage gives you the most benefit with the fewest side effects.

# An Ayurvedic Sexual Wonder Drug

A friend of mine once took a taxi driven by a New York cabdriver who insisted that he was seventy years old, though he looked much younger. His hair was thick and shiny, his complexion glistened, and he bustled with energy. His rejuvenation secret was Chinese ginseng and Shilajit, a moistening Ayurvedic tonic made from bitumen. Shilajit is made up of aluminium, antimony, calcium, cobalt, copper, iron, lithium, magnesium, manganese, molybdenum, phosphorus, silica, sodium, strontium, zinc, fatty acids, hippuric acid, benzoic acid (an antiseptic), fulvic and tannic acids, resin, albuminoids, and glycosides. Studies show it to be effective in treating anemia, liver dysfunction, and muscular atrophy. Allergies are stabilized, and wear and tear on internal organs is reduced by using Shilajit. The recommended dosage is two capsules daily. It is not suitable for people who have kidney stones. Shilajit generates sexual fluids as it clears the body of impurities.

I recommend Shilajit for men and women who live overheated, stressful lives and for those who eat unwisely. This coal by-product feels centering and grounding, and leads energy inward and downward toward the organs of elimination. As we feel rooted, we contact feelings and sensitivity that we normally ignore. Modern life too often inflates us with speed and hot air. We feel scattered, frail, and overcome. Shilajit takes us back to the coal mine to enhance rejuvenation deep in the center of our sexuality. It moistens and rebuilds the sexual organs as it supports adrenal function. That provides needed rest to the adrenal glands so that fewer hormone imbalances occur from fatigue and stress. In India, the herb is recommended for infertility from exhaustion.

# Possible Side Effects of Moistening Tonics

What constitutes overuse of a moistening herb and how can you avoid it? The answer is simple: when you are not thirsty, don't drink. If you don't have vaginal dryness, dry skin, thirst, or other symptoms of dryness, you may not require moistening herbs.

Another possibility is that you need moisturizing but your body can't tolerate other aspects of the remedy. For example, what if your digestion is slow? Moistening herbs can slow digestion even more. Say for example you have bloating, indigestion, or a greasy coating on your tongue, but you still have sexual dryness. What to do then? Combine moistening herbs with others to aid digestion. Ginger, cardamom, dried orange peel, and Chinese ginseng are often used along with the above moistening herbs to ensure absorption without side effects.

# For Women

## Natural Estrogen

Phytoestrogen—the natural estrogen found in plants—can safely help relieve many menopausal symptoms such as hot flashes, insomnia, and vaginal dryness. Natural estrogens do not put you at risk of breast fibroids or other side effects of synthetic hormones.

Among our most commonly used foods containing phytoestrogens are many that also prevent fibroids:

Tofu and soy products

Sunflower seeds

Oats, oat bran, rice bran, wheat germ, rye, barley

Corn, peas, carrots, asparagus, fennel, squash, green bell pepper,
    garlic, sweet potato, onion

Apples, pears, cherries, pomegranates

Beans and legumes

Olive oil

# Health Food Store Phytoestrogen Pills

Lucky for us, several major American health product manufacturers rec-ognize that women need special supplements to ensure health, vitality, and beauty. The Vitamin Shoppe, a chain store with more than thirty locations in New York and New Jersey and accessible by mail order, offers a wide range of health products, including supplements suitable for men and women. I include these Vitamin Shoppe combinations because they present a sensible way to combine necessary vitamins, minerals, and nat-ural hormone herbs.

Estrogen Factors contains vitamins C, E, $B_6$, and $B_3$ along with these natural hormone herbs: Mexican wild yam for progesterone, suma, tang kuei, chaste tree berry *(Vitex agnus castus),* and black cohosh for hormone balance.

Phyto Estrogen Power combines the benefits of soy germ, kudzu root, Korean ginseng, tang kuei, chaste tree berry, and Mexican wild yam, along with vitamin E.

Change-O-Life, made by Nature's Way, contains herbs that balance hormones to ensure a smooth transition to menopause and eliminate most menopausal complaints. They include black cohosh root, sarsaparilla, Siberian ginseng, and phytoestrogenic herbs such as blessed thistle, licorice root, and false unicorn.

# Hormonal Creams for External Use

Various forms of wild yam cream are available, including the Vitamin Shoppe's Progestone-HP and Born Again Wild Yam. These are more than lubricating creams for dry, rough skin. They contain natural diosgenin, a precursor to progesterone, which relieves vaginal dryness and discomfort. Apply a little daily to breasts and sexual area. When used by either sex before lovemaking, a yam cream can enhance pleasurable sensations. These creams have no unpleasant fragrance or side effects.

## The Calcium Issue

I don't have to stress the importance of calcium. Everyone has already told you that it ensures healthy teeth and bones, keeps your heart beating regularly, reduces nervous disorders, and helps you sleep. Calcium absorption is reduced by a diet of excess fat; caffeine; oxalic acid found in chocolate, raw spinach, and rhubarb; and phytic acid found in many grains. Lacking adequate calcium, we suffer the effects of stress, iron deficiency, and brittle bones.

## Natural Calcium Sources

Here are some excellent calcium sources you may not be aware of. The advantage in using vegetable calcium is that plants often contain nutrients necessary for healthy absorption without causing milk allergies.

To protect bones and nerves eat generous amounts of celery, kale, collard greens, turnip greens, broccoli, okra, hijiki, kelp, and dulse seaweeds, almonds, soybeans, tofu, brewer's yeast, corn tortillas with lime added, cooked spinach, parsley, dandelion greens, beet greens, watercress, romaine lettuce, Brazil nuts, walnuts, pecans, peanuts, sunflower seeds, sesame seeds, chickpeas, baked beans, white beans, pinto beans, wheat bran, wheat germ, ripe olives, and dried figs, apricots, raisins, currants, and dates.

Also eat sensible amounts of salmon, mackerel, sardines, canned herring, and tuna with their bones. I also like taking oyster-shell calcium pills and pearl powder sold in Chinese herb shops. Powdered pearl, when added to water, improves your complexion and nerves. Goat's milk and powdered goat whey are excellent sources of natural sodium, necessary for calcium absorption.

One of the most enjoyable sources of vitamin D is sunshine, but the highest source is cooked eel, a Japanese delicacy you can find anywhere that sells sushi. Japanese women are among the longest-lived on the planet. This may be the result of diet, but I suspect it is also influenced by the grace, thoughtfulness, and consideration for others I have enjoyed among my Japanese women friends.

## Calcium Spurs and Bone Disorders

In *Asian Health Secrets* I describe a number of natural painkillers for arthritis such as ArthPlus, made by Nature's Herbs; Mobility 3, made by Health Concerns; and Chinese patent pills, including Guan Jie Yan Wan. Those are remedies after the fact. They help reduce inflammatory pain and swelling by supplementing hormones, increasing circulation, and clearing excess uric acid. However, for extra calcium deposits such as bone spurs, another method works better.

Luckily for us, Chinese doctors have devised successful herbal combinations that address the underlying causes of weak bones. Calcium seeps out of bones when stress, age, caffeine, or illness weakens adrenal glands and disrupts blood production and hormone balance. Old age feels as though we lose vitality through our pores. Skin sags, teeth become loose, and hair falls out because adrenal vitality, which provides stimulation and rhythm to hormone production, slows down. The way to counter this is with nutritious foods and fortifying herbal tonics. (See Letha's Deep-Rejuvenating Serum, page 231.)

Kang Gu Zeng Sheng Pian, made by the Foshanshi Zhiyao Yichang in Guangdong, China, is a kidney-adrenal tonic containing blood-building herbs such as rehmannia and adrenal tonics such as cistanchis and epimedium. In clinical studies done in China involving thousands of people, it proved to be 90 percent effective in treating inflammation of the back and neck vertebrae, degenerative arthritis, bone spurs, and deformed large joints. The formula reduces pain, relieves tense muscles, and strengthens bones while it increases circulation. The best results were seen after three months' use, although severe cases required as much as six months' use. Normal dosage is six pills three times daily (not recommended during a cold or a fever).

# A Ten-Day Plan
# for Menopausal Complaints

*Breakfast:* Hot green tea and a selection of anti-fibroid foods: cabbage, tofu, broccoli, cauliflower, Brussels sprouts, oats, barley, whole wheat, brown rice, ginger, carrots, celery, cucumber, potato, parsnips, onion, chives, garlic, turmeric, citrus fruits, cantaloupe, berries, grapes, mint, oregano, rosemary, sage, thyme, basil, and tarragon. Choose either a fruit or vegetable group each morning and steep the kitchen herbs as teas. Take capsules of dandelion, alfalfa, and weight loss herbs for cleansing, and gotu kola for the nerves as needed.

*10:00 A.M.:* Licorice spice tea or green tea. One hawthorn capsule for circulation. Take vitamins, including B complex, C, A, E, and lecithin.

*Lunch:* A big vegetable salad, steamed rice, and a healthy fish or soup. Take evening primrose oil, calcium, magnesium, and vitamin D, along with Omega 3 fish oils.

*Snack:* Dried apricots or figs, fresh strawberries, or other anti-fibroid fruits or vegetables.

*Dinner:* A delicious meal featuring a healthy protein cooked with aphrodisiac herbs.

*Other:* Long walks, plenty of exercise and rest, daily supplements of natural hormones from plant sources, including one of the following: Change-O-Life or Fem-Mend by Nature's Way, Blessed Thistle Combination by Nature's Herbs, or Restorative Tablets, Women's Harmony, or Menaplex by Health Concerns. Also useful are moistening nonhormonal herbal combinations such as Six Flavor Tea, the Chinese patent remedy also known as Liu Wei Di Huang Wan, and Shou Wu Pien.

# For Men

For information on sexual tonics, please see Chapter 14. The following herbal combinations ensure general vitality and endurance and supply hormone precursors. A healthy trend in health food store supplements combines nutritional supplements such as vitamins, minerals, and amino acids with herbs and other natural rejuvenating substances such as hormones. They all work well together. The body absorbs them better because of the combination. Here are a few examples.

Testosterone Factors, made by The Vitamin Shoppe, contains pantothenic acid, niacin, and vitamins C, D, and B$_6$, along with several amino acids and hormone precursors, including Mexican wild yam, beta sitosterol, frucosterol, campasterol, stigmasterol, and gamma oryzanol, which can stimulate "growth-releasing" hormones. Panax ginseng is added for vitality and good absorption.

Action Max for Men, manufactured by The Vitamin Shoppe, provides a double whammy of protection. Several herbal ingredients, including ashwagandha and yohimbe, have aphrodisiac and tonic properties, while other powerful herbs such as saw palmetto are used for prostate inflammation. To round off the nutritional support, the formula also contains calcium, magnesium, zinc, potassium, and PAK (pyridoxal alpha ketoglutarate), which facilitates the conversion of blood sugar into energy, calms the nerves, and increases oxygen in the tissues. Yohimbe should not be combined with antidepressant medications or alcohol.

# Nutritional Help for Special Problems

I've already written quite a bit about arthritis and fibroids in previous chapters, including diets, supplements, and herbal treatments. Here are a few additional quick prevention tips.

## Arthritis

For daily calcium take a good time-release supplement containing 1,000 mg calcium and 500 mg magnesium along with vitamin D and trace minerals. You need natural sodium-, potassium-, and calcium-rich foods such as black figs and goat's milk (see Bernard Jensen's *Arthritis, Rheumatism, and Osteoporosis*).

Natural sources of calcium include asparagus, Brussels sprouts, cucumber, dandelion, tuna, salmon, and sardines with bones. Seaweeds rich in calcium are hijiki, kelp, and dulse. Of those, kelp is the richest source. Each 100 grams of kelp is equal to 1,093 mg of calcium, which corresponds to ten times more calcium than is found in a comparable amount (3½ oz) of milk. Dulse has three times more calcium than milk and hijiki has fourteen times more.

To help clear congestion try rice cakes or one slice of rye bread spread with a scant amount of prepared horseradish. One-quarter cup of chopped raw white Bermuda onion daily will quickly clear congestion in sinuses and at the joints. Add one-quarter to one-half cup raw red cabbage for painful arthritis. See my Red-Hot Juice for joint pain on page 85. If the pain is inflammatory—if joints are red and burning—omit the horseradish and all hot spices. The juice is very pungent. You may wish to drink it when you won't be around people for a few hours.

Also useful daily for arthritis are ten alfalfa capsules spaced throughout the day, three cod liver oil capsules containing a total of 3,000 IU of vitamin A and 400 IU of vitamin D. Don't forget vitamin C for a total of 3,000 to 8,000 mg of a time-release dosage daily and up to 1,000 mg daily of vitamin E. Don't take the vitamin E at the same time as iron because it will interfere with iron's absorption.

One easy way to do this is to take a time-release pill containing important minerals as well as trace minerals. Metals such as copper, which helps iron absorption, manganese, which maintains a healthy liver, and zinc, which helps blood sugar balance are quite important trace minerals.

Glucosamine has become a popular nutrient used to rebuild damaged joint cartilage. Eric, my chiropractor-bodybuilder brother, says that glucosamine is best absorbed in the stomach when taken with something acidic such as vitamin C or citrus fruits. He recommends three 500 mg capsules with citrus juice three times daily for two weeks, then cut back to half that dose. You will be able to see and feel its effects within three months. You should enjoy a greater range of movement and less pain.

Avoid coffee, black tea, and chocolate because they pull nutrients, including calcium, out of your bones.

# Fibroids

Soy products have wonderful rejuvenative powers. Soy milk and tofu provide healthy natural estrogens while they moisten and nourish the skin, hair, and internal organs. When you combine soy milk with turmeric, a natural antibiotic that enhances circulation and dissolves impurities, you create a healing drink that helps prevent tumors. I recommend one or more glasses of soy milk daily, adding one-half teaspoon of turmeric powder to each glass. If you are constipated, warm the milk and add a handful of Chinese dried apricot kernels for a smooth, satisfying taste and a moistening laxative effect. If you prefer, sweeten with vanilla. This drink will beautify your skin.

To help prevent breast fibroids, give up cigarettes, coffee, black tea, and chocolate. If you are a chocolate freak, try Chyavanprash, a delicious East Indian substitute (see page 112). Green tea is a better choice than coffee because it is digestive, cleansing, slimming, and refreshing. Drink as much hot green tea and peppermint as you like.

Dissolving fibroids takes time, but this recipe works quite well after several months to clear the uterus of extra tissue and the breast of lumps: Twice daily add one-quarter cup aloe vera gel to apple juice, water, or green tea, and take two capsules myrrh and six capsules dandelion. These simple cleansing herbs clear impurities as they dissolve masses. Expect to see clots in your period. Also see the suggestions on page 133.

If you have a sweet tooth but are afraid of putting on weight or increasing fatty tumors from rich sweets, have a healthy digestive remedy for dessert. Papaya and pineapple enzymes are used in Germany as standard fibroid-prevention remedies. When I don't have the fresh fruit at hand, I take a handful of pills. The Vitamin Shoppe makes Papaya Enzyme Plus, which contains papain from papaya melon and leaves and bromelain from pineapple, with no yeast, corn, milk, or other additives. It makes a sweet snack with a cup of tea.

When you think of prevention and treatment not as a tragedy or chore, it becomes part of your pleasure and you feel more protected. Before you put anything into your mouth, think for a moment of what it could become—a boon to beauty and vitality or a problem. Make your health habits part of your everyday life. That way you can keep yourself well, vibrant, and moving forward to seek new adventures. This chapter's tools for building your strength and cooling your nerves can make your fifties and beyond a high-energy, high-productivity, and high-pleasure time of life.

# The Greatest Gift

I recently met the woman called the Queen of Spanish Dance, Pilar Rioja. She's celebrating her twenty-fifth season at the Repertorio Español theater on East Twenty-seventh Street in New York City.

I've had the pleasure of studying with excellent dancers in New York. José Molina is one of my favorites. Another is Andrea Del Conte, an elegant, talented flamenco dancer and a caring teacher. Andrea has attained respect and celebrity, but she is still young for a dance form that respects its senior artists. Pilar Rioja is past sixty and her teacher, Manolo Vargas, is past eighty.

Pilar is petite—a scant five feet tall, weighing one hundred pounds. One critic from Madrid wrote that on stage "she buds forth, she becomes gigantic, she transforms herself, she fills and changes everything; and we begin to become silent, to vanish, to feel that nothing that is not her dancing is of any importance." A statue called the Queen of Spanish Dance was erected in Moscow in her honor after she taught the teachers of the Bolshoi; this amazingly young woman is genuinely sweet and shy, unlike many others dancing to the top.

I stared at her clear, bright skin, uncluttered by makeup, her long dark hair that fell down her back, and her lithe, graceful body. I asked for her rejuvenation secrets. First and foremost, she dances. She has always had "a deep need" to dance. She started at age four but says anyone can dance at any age.

Her teacher, Manolo, started dancing at thirty. Quite handsome and in great shape from dancing flamenco, he has the amusing habit of stopping older people on the street in Mexico City, where he teaches. He asks them their age, then tells them, "I look better than you and am much older." Manolo watches his diet and does yoga and tai chi daily.

Pilar says she stays young because she really knows her body. Her diet is simple. "Only a little white fish, vegetables, but absolutely no bread or sweets," she says. She takes no medicine of any kind. She has refused surgery or painkillers and prefers to exercise pain away. Her performances are two-hour high-energy workouts. When she's not performing, she might dance as many as five hours daily. In the last twenty years, her dancing style has changed, becoming more personal and interior, from the addition of tai chi and yoga. She prefers flamenco to other dance styles because it allows her to be free and expressive and because the footwork and straight posture are good for the body. "You have to pull in your stomach and gluts to look good for flamenco." She stands to demonstrate. "That keeps you young," she says as she strikes a pose. The simplicity of her explanations is refreshing. Her dance is her comfort and companion, her art and her medicine. It is her greatest gift to us and to herself.

## Keys

### Phytoestrogens
Foods: Soy products, especially tofu; raw sunflower and pumpkin seeds, oats, corn, peas, carrots, asparagus, apples, squash, beans, olive oil, royal jelly, and bee pollen
Herbs: Blessed thistle, false unicorn, cohosh, fo-ti
Vitamin Shoppe: Estrogen Factors, Phyto-Estrogen Power
Nature's Way: Change-O-Life

### Testosterone
Herbs: Epimedium, high-dose Siberian ginseng
Vitamin Shoppe: Testosterone Factors, Action Max for Men

### Calcium sources
Kelp, kale, collard greens, broccoli, hijiki, dulse, okra, endive

### Heart trouble prevention
Anticholesterol: green tea, hawthorn
Angina: raw tienchi ginseng (page 240)

**Links:** Also see Chapters 4, 6, 8, 11, 13–17

# PART FOUR

# ENERGY, VITALITY, AND SEXUALITY

*The spark of life and light is your destiny.*

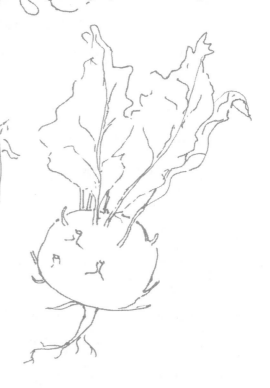

The spark of life given you will not fail if you listen to your body and use herbs. Do not save pleasure for the future. Live full out, but protect your vitality with the right herbs, foods, and mental clarity.

In your healing space, observe your tongue in a mirror.

Is your tongue pale? Is your vitality low? Do you suffer chills, depression, lethargy, poor concentration, or fatigue? Do your lower back and legs ache? Do you need to urinate frequently? Has your sexual fire gone out? If so, you require warming tonic herbs such as Chinese ginseng, ginger, cloves, cardamom, sage, and thyme. Warming herbal tonics enhance energy, muscle tone, breathing, and physical endurance. Warm, nourishing cooked meals and the company of loving friends will comfort you.

Is your tongue red and dry? Do you frequently feel nervous, fearful, or anxious? Do you get fever, night sweats, or hot flashes? Are you irritable too often? Is it hard to stay asleep at night? Are you often thirsty? Do you smoke or use hot spices, garlic, or caffeine? Do you have dry skin and premature gray hair? If so, you require moistening, cooling foods and herbs such as asparagus, oatmeal, almonds, American ginseng, tofu, and green vegetables. Cooling, moistening tonics enhance beauty, patience, and depth of feelings. Knowing this, you can nurture yourself better than any parent can.

# CHAPTER 13

# Total Energy for Work and Play

*Age means nothing: energy is everything.*

---

*Your Goal:* **To find specific causes and cures for physical and mental exhaustion.**

*Materials:* **These will vary depending upon which of the five elements are involved. The fire element requires heart stimulant and digestive herbs. The earth element requires herbs that maintain healthy blood sugar balance and a cheerful mood. The metal element requires remedies that facilitate breathing and elimination of toxins. The water element requires herbs that build immunity to illness and enliven sexual vitality, and the wood element thrives on herbs that ensure muscle strength and flexibility. Exhaustion can result from a weakness in any of these.**

---

Watching our cat, Silky, play with her ball, I see her muscles tense as she prepares to spring. She is liquid energy in motion. Charging, she overshoots and gracefully somersaults over the ball. Nonchalant, she stands up to stretch. I've never seen her act tired. When it's nap time, she naps. People should be as wise as cats.

You may know why you are tired, but it's more complicated than you think. Vitality runs down in many ways. There are wonderful herbs for each cause of fatigue. Please answer a few questions to determine the origin of *your* exhaustion. Herbal help can be found at the end of each section. Which sections—fire, earth, metal, water, or wood—have you checked most often? Compare your answers with the five element energy types in Chapter 4.

# Fire

—When I'm tired I feel it in my heart or chest.

—I'm often tired in the mornings.

—Hard work makes my heartbeat irregular.

—I have high LDL cholesterol.

—I feel tired when I'm emotional or sentimental.

—I laugh and talk a lot.

—I love to express my feelings.

—I wake up at night with heart palpitations.

—I've had heart trouble.

—I'm overweight or enjoy eating rich foods.

—I drink coffee.

—I have thyroid problems.

—I feel chest pains when under stress.

—I often look flushed or blush easily.

—I get sores in my mouth when I overwork.

—I can't sleep when I'm upset or overtired.

—I take stimulant drugs or medicine.

—I thrive on speed and excitement.

—I enjoy the taste of bitter drinks such as coffee and tea.

—When I perspire or have a fever, my odor smells slightly burned.

The fire element is associated with the heart, pericardium, small intestine, and an acupuncture meridian involved with both temperature and metabolism called the triple heater. When the fire element is unbalanced by stress or fatigue, circulation, memory, and emotions will be affected. A fire person can frequently be exhausted by intense emotions or overuse of stimulants. But anyone can have a problem with the fire element from overwork and extreme worry. Fatigue affects the fire element when you feel it in your heart.

## Tired Weak Heart and Fatigue

The best remedy for chronic fatigue affecting heart rhythm, mental clarity, and memory is one that makes the heart act normally such as hawthorn. Hawthorn berries, sold in health food store capsules, are a gentle stimulant for tired heart muscles. They reduce cholesterol and make your heart stronger, ensuring the brain's blood supply. Hawthorn is an excellent herb for high-stress executives or anyone under constant pressure. In most cases you'll get relief from chest pain and fatigue in a week or two by taking one capsule of hawthorn after meals.

A Chinese hospital study with 470 patients proved Qi Zhi Ling oral liquid to be effective for memory, mental focus, Alzheimer's disease, and insomnia. It contains polygonum, polygola, jujube, mulberry, wolfberry, and ginseng.

## Rapid Heart Palpitations and Panic

Heart irregularities can aggravate anxiety and vice versa. If you lie awake at night worrying or awaken suddenly in heart-pounding alarm, you need a remedy that soothes the heart such as homeopathic gelsemium 30c (yellow jasmine). It is recommended for anxiety about future events. Often taking one dose of it makes you feel as though the butterflies in your stomach have landed.

Physical exhaustion or overweight makes the heart work overtime. If you have those problems, you need herbs that won't threaten energy or impair the body's ability to deal with excess cholesterol. You may have to use digestive remedies if your heartbeat feels irregular after rich eating.

Ding Xin Wan is a Chinese patent remedy designed to enhance and balance our deepest sources of vitality—the heart and adrenal glands. It is most often recommended for insomnia. Too often when adrenal strength is exhausted, our lower back aches, we have heart palpitations, anxiety, and restlessness as well as poor memory and concentration. A harmonizing remedy such as Ding Xin Wan brings things back into order because it helps vitality without sedating energy. When you are overwrought and can't sleep, taking a heart-balancing remedy can actually improve energy and concentration the next day because it supports vitality.

In extreme cases, homeopathic aconite 30c treats panic, restlessness, and fear of death and crowds. Persons who need homeopathic aconite are overly sensitive to light, noise, and touch.

Heart-healthy foods also reduce excess cholesterol and strengthen blood vessels, while ensuring their flexibility. They include five to ten cups of green tea with peppermint daily; oatmeal; oat bran and vegetable fiber sources; fruits and vegetables; tofu; grape-seed extract, red wine (page 50), and Omega 3 fish oils. Taking daily doses of niacin (niacinamide, or vitamin B$_3$) and mixed trace minerals helps ensure healthy circulation. If your heart and blood vessels are clear of plaque and resilient to shocks, you will have better energy and mental capacity and will live longer.

# Earth

—I feel tired after eating a meal.

—If I don't eat regularly, I feel weak and spacey.

—I crave sweets and enjoy pastry or cookies for dessert.

—I call my honey sweet nicknames.

—When I argue, I get a stomachache.

—I am a faithful and loyal friend.

—My waistline is a bit too large.

—My fatigue is worse during late afternoon.

—When tired, I get hungry.

—I am diabetic or have diabetic relatives.

—My hypoglycemia makes me moody.

—I love going to great restaurants.

—I devour books, movies, and other pleasures.

—I sit at a desk all day.

—Humid weather tires me.

—I like to tell jokes and be the life of the party.

—My home is my castle.

—Changing jobs or relationships throws me off center.

—When upset I get diarrhea.

—I often have a stomachache.

The digestive energy of the earth element affects the stomach and spleen-pancreas, seen as one organ in traditional Chinese medicine. If you feel off center from stress, overeating, or a blood sugar imbalance, you may experience fatigue, spaciness, lethargy, and depression. Earth energy is challenged by rich eating and emotional upset. It's because our earth, the digestive center, is also our emotional center.

## Indigestion, Blood Sugar, and Energy

The best remedies for anyone who loves to eat richly at irregular hours—or who finds comfort in food, stable relationships, and an unvarying routine—are those that fortify the digestive center. Do you like to eat the same thing every day? Or at the same time? Does your routine give you a sense of security? Emotional comfort and good digestion are earth issues.

Xiao Yao Wan is an excellent traditional Chinese herbal combination for earth types or people addicted to junk foods, stress, and obsessive tendencies. It treats hypoglycemia, indigestion, and depression. It's a great little pill remedy for sweet, cuddly writers chained to their chairs or for anyone else who chews on problems all day.

Xiao Yao Wan contains digestive herbs such as ginger, mint, bupleurum; blood-building herbs, including tang kuei, paeonia root, and atractylodes; and poria, a mild diuretic. If you have a pale tongue, indicating slow metabolism, this remedy will lift your energy immediately. If, on the other hand, you have a dry red tongue from dehydration or a speedy metabolism, this remedy will not be as effective. If you have an ulcer or excess acid, avoid this remedy and use aloe vera gel instead.

## Ulcer Burn and Energy

It's hard to concentrate when you are in pain. Excess digestive acid can scatter your attention unless you take the right herbs. Aloe vera is a very alkaline healing plant. It mends burned skin from sunburn or scalding. Taken internally in juice, it heals ulcer burns. Add one-half cup of aloe juice or gel, available in health food stores, to apple or other juice once or twice daily. Aloe is slightly laxative, which is very helpful for anyone with a red tongue. Daily doses of zinc and chromium are important for digestive health and blood sugar balance.

When digestive energy is smooth and strong, you'll feel stable, confident, and happy to be in your emotional center. The world will be a lovely place, and you will be able to continue digesting—words, ideas, relationships, or whatever—in peace.

# Metal

—I'm tired because I can't breathe.

—Walking up the stairs takes my breath away.

—I feel pale and listless.

—I smoke or I used to smoke.

—Sometimes I cough a lot.

—I have asthma, emphysema, tuberculosis, or cystic fibrosis.

—I am a great collector—art, clothes, you name it.

—I often feel weepy and sad.

—I get sinus infections or often feel stuffed up.

—I had terrible acne as a kid, or I still have it.

—I frequently get constipated or have diarrhea.

—I have skin blemishes or blotches.

—I have numerous addictions.

—The world is closing in on me.

—I hold grudges.

—I can't perspire, or I perspire too often.

—My lungs feel congested.

—I crave hot, sweet, and sour foods.

—I have deformed joints.

—When I fight, I am as tough as steel.

The energy dynamic of the metal element involves our relationship to others and to the space around us. The metal element in traditional Chinese medicine is made up of the lungs and large intestine. When the metal element is healthy, we have deep breath and adequate oxygen that ensure proper energy and mental focus. Our relationship to space—our surroundings—is also healthy. If the metal element is damaged by illness or bad habits, however, we cannot inhale and exhale properly. We feel cramped and without air in our space. We feel as though the world is closing in on us.

## Shortness of Breath and Low Energy

People weakened by shallow breath lack stamina. They isolate themselves in order to save their energy. Consequently their relationships to others suffer. They may feel so isolated that they engage in dangerous addictions such as drugs and smoking to shut out the world. The voice of a depressed person is often shallow, gasping, or ungrounded. Such people lack strength and assurance. The best remedies for people who have difficulty breathing, those who work in toxic environments, or people who feel shut in are herbs that improve breathing.

## Warming Herbs for Weakness and Wheezing

Thyme, sage, clove, ginger, and basil are useful for people with shortness of breath, weakness, and wheezing asthma. Make sure you have a pale tongue before using any of these herbs or teas, which are drying and inflammatory. They are strong energy stimulants.

## Cooling Herbs for Panting and Thirst

If you are fatigued and short of breath but have a red tongue, you will have a hard time catching your breath. Inflammation in the lungs dries oxygen fast. Avoid all hot spices, pungent foods such as radishes, and drying foods such as popcorn. All inflammatory foods will feel irritating. Instead, you need cooling, moisturizing herbs that increase saliva and fluids, such as American ginseng tea. Unlike Chinese ginseng, American ginseng is moisturizing and soothing for people with chronic fever conditions and dry cough or for people who smoke. Drink lots of it if you have any of those conditions.

Other moistening foods beneficial for the lungs are asparagus, almonds, and oatmeal. (Also see my recipes for beautiful skin in Chapter 5.) When the right herbs heal your lungs, your breathing capacity will enlarge. The added oxygen intake will improve both your energy and your concentration, and it will beautify your skin. Alternating doses of homeopathic ferrum phos. 6x (iron) and homeopathic kali. sulph. 6x (potassium) five times throughout the day will add oxygen and vibrancy to your skin.

# Water

—I have dark circles or bags under my eyes.

—I moan or groan when I speak.

—My complexion has a grayish cast.

—I am tired most of the time, but especially in the afternoon.

—Sometimes I can't sleep all night and feel tired the next day.

—I live several lives at once, working and playing all the time.

—I can't let down one minute. I have to do everything myself.

—My back aches!

—I urinate too frequently or not often enough.

—My sexual enthusiasm is very high.

—My sexual energy needs help.

—I am overweight.

—My ankles are swollen or puffy.

—I love salty and spicy foods.

—I have had cancer or other immune-threatening diseases.

—I have high cholesterol or blood pressure problems.

—Everything tires me.

—I could sleep all the time.

—I prefer spectator sports to any sort of exercise.

—Let the world take care of itself.

The water element is said to "contain" the kidney and bladder energies. The kidney, in Chinese medicine, includes its entire energy system—the adrenal glands, hormones, the brain and its brain chemicals along with the biorhythms that affect it. If your water element is challenged by overwork, jet lag, illness, or medication, your energy is bound to suffer.

## Adrenal Weakness and Chronic Fatigue

Most people living stressful lives have some of the above symptoms of weak adrenal energy, and they need to know how to rebuild their vitality. After a long period of abuse, rest is not enough. The best remedies for people who have long-term chronic fatigue are complicated herbal remedies that nourish both blood production and energy capacity.

Compound GL, made by Seven Forests, is an herbal treatment for chronic fatigue syndrome. A number of my clients swear by it. Following the directions on the bottle, they took the pills over a period of two weeks to two months and reported a remarkable improvement in vitality, mental concentration, and endurance. The formula contains many blood and energy tonic herbs. You or your health food store can order it from a number of the distributors listed in the Herbal Access section at the back of the book.

## Low Energy Means Low Immune Strength

Tonic herbs do more than improve energy; they also enhance the basic elements of vibrant good health, including strong immunity to illness. Since alternative medicine stresses prevention, many excellent products are available among Eastern and Western herbal traditions.

I prefer Asian medicine because it is by nature more specific. Herbal choice applies more directly to an individual person. There is no one herbal quick-fix remedy that works for everybody in the same way. To best use this ancient healing tradition, you have to get to know yourself by observing your symptoms. Here are two examples of kidney energy tonics that work in different ways. The first is warming; the second is cooling and moisturizing.

Sexoton and Liu Wei Di Huang Wan are Chinese patent remedies I have already discussed. Use Sexoton if you have wheezing, watery diarrhea, and frequent urination. Use the second one if you need a moisturizing tonic because you have problems such as dry cough, night sweats, or constipation. Taking herbs to rebuild adrenal and kidney energy gives you a new lease on life. It enhances your immunity to disease and fortifies the glue that holds you together—your blood, bone marrow, and endurance.

# Wood

—I get tired from fighting with people.
—I like everything in its place.
—I find it hard to make up my mind.
—When I get upset, I feel enraged or nauseated.
—I have a bad temper.
—I enjoy hot spicy food and exciting people.
—I love to travel.
—When I can't travel or carry out my plans, I feel very frustrated.
—Sometimes my skin has a jaundiced or coppery tone.
—I can't sleep when I get excited.
—I don't tire or get sick unless I'm upset.
—Rich and greasy foods make me sick.
—Incompetence makes me angry.
—I have allergies, headaches, or gout.
—I am getting arthritis, or my joints hurt in humid weather.
—My skin is dry and cracked.
—I love to exercise, dance, or work out in a gym.
—I strive for perfection.
—I like to lead the pack.
—I get muscle spasms, or my muscle tone needs improving.

The dynamic of the wood element is movement. Its internal organs, the liver and gallbladder, affect digestion, circulation, the absorption of calcium, and the strength and agility of muscles. If the wood element is challenged by rich diet or conflicting emotions, vision also suffers. That is because muscles affecting vision are subject to circulation, which, in turn, is affected by calcium. Most people with wood problems are nearsighted or have an astigmatism.

## Toxins and Fatigue

If the body is struggling to rid itself of environmental or dietary impurities, it has less energy left over for everything else. People who demand the most and best from themselves most often do not take time to chew each mouthful of food twenty times and brush after every meal. People who develop wood problems may eat richly and worry more about their work than about their health.

## Bitter Cleansing Herbs

Since the wood element is intimately linked with the liver and, therefore, with our ability to rid the body of toxins, the best remedies for wood problems are those that cleanse the body of impurities. They are bitter laxative and diuretic herbs, including aloe vera, dandelion, skullcap, gentian, burdock, alfalfa, and cascara sagrada.

If you have constipation or skin blemishes, dandelion, burdock, and cascara sagrada, a laxative, will help you. If you have irritability, insomnia, or hot flashes, skullcap will cool and cleanse the liver. If you have arthritis, alfalfa and yucca will be beneficial. If you have spaciness, chronic diarrhea, and depression, gentian extract will balance you. These bitter, cleansing herbs can help your energy because they improve the functioning of the liver. If you have a healthy liver, fewer irritants and allergens will bother you.

Persons with wood problems—those who love to exercise their minds, willpower, and muscles—suffer the fatigue that comes from excess activity or drive. Sometimes, when desires and aspirations cannot be met, they are exhausted from frustration. They can be helped with herbs that soothe, build, and cleanse the liver. To soothe and cleanse the liver use aloe vera. Drink one-half cup daily in apple juice to improve irritability, constipation, joint pain, and nervousness.

## Liver-Building Herbs

Blood tonics such as he shou wu, which is sold in health food stores as foti, and the Chinese patent remedy Liu Wei Di Huang Wan are helpful to rebuild a damaged liver. They are very moisturizing and not digestive. If you suffer from indigestion from rich or heavy foods, take these moisturizing tonics with a digestive herb such as ginger or cardamom. Having adequate blood will improve your energy and outlook.

## Liver Repair after Fever, Illness, and Addiction

Another useful herb to rebuild a liver damaged by chemicals, drugs, illness, or alcohol is *Eclipta prostrata*—in Chinese, han lian cao. The dried plant is sweet, sour, and cooling in quality. You can order eclipta by mail as a powder and add it to capsules. Take six to eight daily if you suffer from cirrhosis of the liver, poor bone marrow, dizziness, and blurred vision associated with blood deficiency.

Eclipta also treats beauty problems associated with liver damage such as hair loss and fragile fingernails and hair. The renewed moisture and reduced water retention will give your health and spirits a boost.

## Energy and Rage

If you can't move forward because of rage, you have to cleanse your liver more carefully. I recommend Lung Tan Xie Gan Wan, a Chinese patent remedy useful for herpes, nervousness, rage, and PMS. Men and women both can use it. Up the dosage from ten to twenty at a time, three times daily, depending on your discomfort level. If you become weak from cleansing or have a pale tongue, combine Lung Tan Xie Gan Wan with Sexoton or Xiao Yao Wan.

Eliminating anger and toxins removes obstructions to self-actualization. You are on your way to making your own perfection. Keeping your energy clear, strong, and balanced can make that possible.

## Combinations and Variations in the Elements

Each of us will pass through symptoms associated with the five elements. Whether you are a water person or not, sooner or later you will suffer from jet lag and exhaustion. Even if you are not a wood person, you may still get a cramp, a headache from arguing, or an allergy. You may feel frustrated—no matter what your element—if you can't move about freely or see the fruits of your imagination come into being. The important thing is to recognize what energy has been weakened and to act accordingly.

# A Five-Day Plan to Balance the Five Elements

This program builds vitality by treating individual problems. Choose a diet to enhance energy and breathing that is made up of easy-to-digest, nutritious foods and pungent spices. Drink hot green tea daily with one slice of raw ginger, fresh mint and tarragon, and aloe vera gel. People with poor digestion, spaciness, shortness of breath, and mucus congestion (see the anti-candida diet, page 155) should eat antioxidant foods, including red peppers, grape-seed extract, and clean vegetable proteins. Use herbs and supplements for weight loss, heart health, and digestion, including B vitamins, zinc, chromium, and trace minerals. For diarrhea, add gentian extract. Between meals choose one or more of the following health food products. See the Herbal Access section for addresses. This questionnaire will help you determine the best tonic for you. If you check several items, you can combine the suggested remedies during the same day.

—"I eat too many salty and sweet foods and stimulants."
   Vrrooom Power or Digestive Harmony from Health Concerns
—"I eat or drink too much, and I feel out of sorts."
   Homeopathic nux vomica 30c

—"I have digestive pain or ulcers."

Bupleurum S and Bupleurum 12 from Health Concerns; aloe vera gel, cumin, raw cabbage juice, and vitamin U

—"I am depressed and have hypoglycemia. I feel shaky or spacey if I don't eat."

Xiao Yao Wan Chinese patent remedy; or ginger, mint, tarragon, parsley, turmeric, chromium, zinc, and trace minerals; anti-candida diet (page 155) and homeopathic carbo veg. 30c; homeopathic pulsatilla 30c for mucus congestion

—"My back hurts. I feel weak and out of breath."

Sexoton, a Chinese patent remedy; or fo-ti capsules along with clove tea; damiana capsules taken in midafternoon

—"I'm tired because I think too much."

Ashwagandha powder added to tea or taken in capsules; Emperors Restoration, Ginseng Root Compound, Nourish, or Two Tigers from Nutritional Life Support Systems; Ginsengs of the World or Ginseng 6 Restorative Caps from Crystal Star; Siberian, American, and Chinese ginseng, gotu kola, royal jelly, and fo-ti; Qi Zhi Ling oral drink (from Lin Sisters)

# Keys

*Pale tongue*—indicating weakness and slow metabolism: Use warming tonic herbs such as Chinese ginseng, sage, ginger, and clove. Of these warming herbs, the following stimulants are best according to your element:

Fire (weak heart, depression): Rosemary, hawthorn, lavender

Earth (indigestion, depression): Ginger, cardamom, kava kava

Metal (shortness of breath, wheezing): Radish, thyme, clove

Water (backache with weakness): Clove, epimedium

Wood (low vitality and enthusiasm): Garlic, ginger, pepper, parsley, alfalfa

*Dry red tongue*—indicating dehydration or fever: Use cooling, moistening herbs and spices such as American ginseng, almonds, oatmeal, and salad greens. Of the cooling remedies, the following are best according to your element:

Fire (fever): Homeopathic ferrum phos.

Earth (stomach ulcer): Cumin, aloe vera gel

Metal (dry cough): American ginseng tea

Water (dark urine): Cilantro, sarsaparilla capsules

Wood (allergies, headache, anger): aloe vera, Lung Tan Xie Gan Wan (see page 120)

## Links: Also see Chapters 6, 8, 10, 16, 17

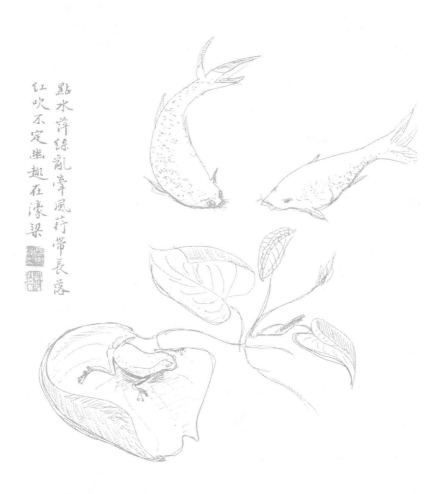

CHAPTER 14

# Sexual Sparks

*It's a bird. It's a plane. It's super you!*

---

*Your Goal:* **To rekindle the flame of love and passion.**

*Materials:* **Vitamin E and zinc; homeopathic gold and silver for sexual power and juice; herbs that replenish semen and moisten dryness, including he shou wu; safe herbal aphrodisiacs. Ginkgo to facilitate circulation. A tea made with epimedium and lycium fruit, which rejuvenates from the bone marrow to the skin's surface. Homeopathic remedies for emotional blocks. Optional: a red cape.**

---

The Superman comics and television programs we grew up watching are synonymous with a great American sexual myth—"faster than a speeding bullet, more powerful than a locomotive." The part of this fairy tale—created by two teenage nerds from Cleveland in the 1930s—that we accept is: you can give it all you've got at work and still be superhuman after hours. Fortunately, tonic foods and herbs can give you energy to work hard and still have drive, power, and juice to fly high in romance.

This chapter is all about the joys of sex and sensuality—the pleasure of being in your body. No matter what your personal persuasion, sexual plenty is essential for a satisfying life. Ample desire as well as abundant sexual hormones maintain youth and beauty even if you fly alone. To stimulate those hormones is in itself rejuvenating.

Testosterone and estrogen, necessary for both sexes, fluctuate throughout life depending on age, exercise habits, and diet. They fuel vitality and intelligence while reducing many discomforts associated with illness and aging, including overweight, arthritic pain, depression,

and menstrual irregularity. In this chapter we will increase sexual pleasure with fortifying herbs and foods that enhance depth of feeling as well
as energy. We will learn to use massage for rejuvenation and as a pre-
lude to joyful sex.

Older men and women tend to resemble each other. This is partly
from a reduction in rejuvenating hormones. Men with reduced testosterone levels become sluggish, develop rounded curves, breasts, and fea-
tures softened by overweight. They may seem uninterested in sex or any
physical activity. Women, whose testosterone levels frequently increase
after menopause, become flushed and aggressive. Some cut their hair to
look like helmets and bark orders at their spouse or co-workers. Romance
can break down over the years, but a genuine lack of sexual responsiveness by either sex has deeper roots.

It is generally recognized that men produce more testosterone and
women more estrogen, giving them sexual differences. Testosterone,
because it raises metabolism level, gives both sexes hard muscles, a lean
body, facial hair, and a deeper voice. Synthetic male hormones make you
irritable and hyperactive and can lead to fibroids. Estrogen increases body
fat, sexual fluids, and breast size. It regulates menstruation and mood
swings, making you feel mellow.

Hormones used as food additives, medicines, or nutritional supplements have unhealthy side effects most people are unaware of. Increased
male sex hormones lead to menstrual and emotional problems and fibroids
for women. Some experts believe that high estrogen levels increase the
likelihood of fatty tumors, breast fibroids, and prostate swelling.

Herbs that safely increase natural hormones have been used in Asia as
an excellent way of maintaining youthfulness because they are combined
in ways that reduce harmful side effects. For example, traditional Chinese
herb doctors combine plant sources of testosterone such as dried
epimedium leaf with blood-building herbs to treat impotence and infertility in either sex, improve heart function, and strengthen lower back and
legs, without increasing facial hair or a martial personality. (See page 231
for Letha's Deep-Rejuvenating Serum for men and women, containing
epimedium.)

This is possible because Asian formulas are not merely aphrodisiacs but include tonic herbs that rebuild sexuality weakened by overwork, worry, or sexual excess. As I've noted, certain moistening herbs are frequently combined in sexual tonics because they increase sexual fluids—semen and vaginal fluid—without affecting estrogen, making them perfect rejuvenation herbs for either sex.

The sexual tonics covered in this chapter are separated into categories for men and women according to their needs. Some herbs apply to both sexes. All the formulas are safe and effective because they encourage proper circulation and healthy adrenal strength. They contain neither animal products nor irritants that increase nervousness.

# The Anatomy of Sexual Energy

According to a classical Chinese medical view, sexual vitality originates with the water element. Sexual *desire* springs from the healthy wood element, made up of the liver and gallbladder energies along with their acupuncture pathways. The wood and water elements' acupuncture meridians—forming the anatomy of sexual desire—direct our vitality through the inner legs to the groin. The liver meridian passes through the sexual organs to the chest and the eyes on its way to the brain. Thus vitality is eventually spread throughout the nervous system and muscles. The wood element facilitates healthy circulation, muscle tone, coordinated movement, clear vision, and a peaceful and strong "soul"—the desire and the ability to actualize our will, to carry through with our dreams.

This does not mean that people with high sexual desire are more often willful or bossy. Willfulness can be a product of unproductive nervous energy. True vitality—and passion—can be seen in the eyes, complexion, and body movements.

Our desire for sex, or any engaging activity, is dampened by poor circulation resulting from rich diet, difficult emotions, or poor habits. Because they clear the liver of impurities and help its action, bitter and pungent digestive herbs improve circulation, mood, and ultimately sexual vitality. Put another way: to have a satisfying sex life, we need strong muscles and good blood circulation.

Sexual pleasure requires circulation to warm our sexual areas. Several popular aphrodisiac herbs do little more than engorge the sexual organs with blood. These herbs can cause problems because they create a physical capacity for sex without enhancing a loving mood. Instead of relying on sexual stimulants such as yohimbe, which have unpleasant side effects, it is wiser to reinforce vitality with aphrodisiacs that maintain sexual health, for example, ginkgo and panax ginseng.

Adrenal energy, originating from the water element, makes sex possible by furnishing hormones. Healthy adrenal glands give us strength in the lower back, legs, and sexual organs. For sex to be physically satisfying, we need adequate strength and sexual hormones as well as smooth circulation. To ensure this, we need to carefully regulate diet, stress levels, emotions, and sexual practices. It is wise to avoid having sex when you are sick, menstruating, or too tired. Instead, choose a fortifying herbal tonic and rest until you feel stronger. Here are a few other recommendations for enhancing desire and pleasure.

- Flirt—It's good for your hormones.
- Wear a fragrance to bed that excites you. Green apple, vanilla, and lavender are calming; rosemary, geranium, and clove stimulate.
- Cook a great meal with aphrodisiac herbs and eat dessert in bed.
- Massage each other's feet with raw sesame oil before retiring.
- Get to bed early and, repair your health with plenty of sleep.

# Diet for Joyful Sex

## Avoid Caffeine

Although at one time considered an aphrodisiac, coffee is one of the worst offenders for circulation. Black tea and chocolate also inhibit circulation, but coffee gets muscle tension stuck in a ball in your chest. It can aggravate hiatal hernia, when tense stomach muscles press against the diaphragm, causing extreme pain. In short, coffee inhibits blood flow to the sexual area. (It leads to short sex.) Coffee can make you hyper because it overstimulates the nervous system, adrenal glands, and heart. It's much healthier to drink green tea with mint. To free stuck circulation, add up to one-quarter teaspoon turmeric powder to a cup of hot tea. To make any tea an aphrodisiac, add a pinch of clove powder to each cup. Clove is a heating herb not meant for people with fevers or dark-colored urine.

## Indigestion and Sex

Digestive herbs free sexual desire and energy because they strengthen the heart and free circulation. Besides, slow digestion can ruin a romantic evening. To avoid frustration, add these to your cooking: ginger, black pepper, mint, cardamom, clove, parsley, tarragon, onions, garlic, and turmeric powder. To heal a weak, irregular heart and slow metabolism, follow meals with one capsule of hawthorn along with a cup of hot ginger tea. Avoid creamy, rich, and fried foods, especially when followed by gooey sweets, otherwise your night of love will be spent painfully digesting. Also see Chapters 9 and 10, regarding weight loss.

## Nutritional Supplements and Sex

The short path to sexual vitality includes generous amounts of certain vitamins and minerals. They may not give you an edge on romance, but they can certainly spark a well-laid fire.

Vitamin E and ginkgo are essential. They free circulation, ward off fatigue, and keep you young. Wheat germ oil, a natural source of E, helps its absorption. Take 400 to 1,000 units daily. Take ginkgo between meals, six or more capsules daily.

Zinc (100 mg daily) can help prevent prostate trouble. It is naturally found in its highest concentration in the prostate. Lack of this nutrient can produce testicle atrophy.

Also remember to take daily B complex tablets; 2,000 to 5,000 mg of vitamin C with bioflavanoids; vitamins A and D; and mixed minerals.

The trace mineral gold is especially helpful for rebuilding tired adrenal glands. An old East Indian rejuvenation secret is to eat rich Indian sweets covered with gold and silver leaf papers. In India, you actually eat the paper. Gold is said to further brilliance, and silver to increase endurance. I prefer taking homeopathic gold (aurum 6x) and homeopathic silver (argentum nit. 6x). Add a dose of each to a cup of spring water and sip it between meals. It puts a precious-metal zing into your walk.

## Nervousness and Sex

Work stress, anger, frustration, and nervousness interfere with love. Try creating a loving atmosphere in your healing space or bedroom. During the workday you can prepare for the evening with nerve-replenishing foods—black cherry, leafy greens, and oatmeal.

Saffron, gotu kola, and a combination of Siberian and American ginseng will soothe emotions without reducing sexual appetite. Add a pinch of saffron to a cup of green tea or water to reduce liver irritation from spicy cooking. If you are sensitive to hot spices and angry emotions, using bitter cleansing herbs such as aloe vera and dandelion daily will be very beneficial.

Between meals you can heal brain fatigue and nervous stress with six capsules daily of gotu kola. It improves concentration. Extracts of Siberian and American ginseng work well together to replenish nerves, brain, and spinal fluid. Use ten drops of each in a cup of water once daily between meals. After your nerves have healed, you will find that Siberian ginseng, a source of testosterone, can act as a stimulant. You may have to adjust the dosage down to reduce nervous insomnia. Men can take more than women. Stop taking Siberian ginseng if it gives you a headache, nervousness, or insomnia.

## Preparation for Love

Two sources of sexual vitality are important. One is the slow, judicious energy and nutrition built daily with a wise diet and herbal supplements.

The other sort of sexual stimulant builds desire and strength in the short term—say, for the evening. I'll cover both with equal consideration because they are both essential. For best results, combine the following products with lovingly prepared healthy meals, soothing music, healing incense, and the sexual massage described on page 231.

# Herbs for Increased Sexual Hormones and Fluids

These foods stimulate the body's natural production of sexual hormones and fluids for men and women: tofu, asparagus, and licorice, damiana, or sarsaparilla tea are estrogenic and rejuvenating. Siberian ginseng can increase testosterone when taken in large dosages suitable for body-builders. Herbal combinations recommended for menopausal discomforts were covered in Chapter 12. The following herbs increase sexual fluids, without affecting hormones, and can be taken as pills, cooked as broth, or served as an herbal wine.

Chinese he shou wu *(Polygonum multiflori),* commonly called fo-ti when sold in health food stores, is a moistening, blood-building herb recommended to stop premature graying of hair, dry skin, and dry cough. It increases sexual fluids for men and women. In Chinese herb shops you will find pills called Shou Wu Pien, which can be ordered from addresses in the back of this book. The normal dosage is five pills three time daily between meals.

If you like to prepare your own herbal brew, cook one handful of sliced he shou wu, a slightly bittersweet herb in a quart of spring water for twenty minutes and drink the decoction warm with a pinch of salt. The prepared medicinal wine, called Shou Wu Chih, sometimes contains 100 percent *Polygonum multiflori* or may contain other blood-tonic herbs such as Chinese angelica. One shot glass, taken at least one hour after the evening meal, is a tasty, relaxing way to recover from chronic sexual exhaustion, childbirth, menopause, or anemia.

Most people are so tired that the semisweet liquor puts them to sleep the first time or two they drink it. Over a period of a few weeks the moistening, restorative effects will pay off: women will enjoy added sexual comfort and men will benefit from having more semen.

# Recommended for Men

Chinese ginseng stimulates nitric oxide and is safer than Viagra. A number of popular tonics, widely available in health food stores, have suggestive names such as Male Performance. They usually include both blood and energy tonic herbs. One example of a general tonic is Male Formula, made by McZand Herbal in Santa Monica. It combines American and Chinese ginseng, fo-ti, and quite a few other herbs, including damiana, sarsaparilla, gotu kola, and skullcap. The formula supplements hormones without giving a sudden jolt of sexual desire or energy. It is meant to keep men healthy, balanced, and strong. That kind of tonic actually builds resistance to illness and depression as much as reducing stress. It's important not to lose sight of the picture—healthy people enjoy healthy sex.

The Vitamin Shoppe manufactures a line of herbal and natural vitamin supplements suited for men's sexual issues. They include Testosterone Factors, which combines necessary vitamins with hormone precursors such as Mexican wild yam and oryzanol, and high-energy herbs.

Several yohimbé products contain the extract of that African tree bark used as an aphrodisiac. They are called Yohimbe 2000, Super Male-Plex, and Sumba Forte. *Beware of products containing yohimbé.* Many people feel its sexual benefits are not worth the possible dangerous side effects. It is an aphrodisiac for men that engorges peripheral blood vessels, making and maintaining an erection—sometimes long after it is desired. It increases neither desire nor love, and it can become a nuisance. Yohimbé should be avoided completely by anyone who is unstable or depressed or who has circulation or blood pressure problems. Its stimulant and depressant components can drive a person over the edge emotionally. Never mix it with antidepressant medications or alcohol.

Some male sexual tonic pills from Chinatown are also hard-hitting in their effects, which can be summed-up as "We want good sex now!" I do not recommend such pills, which are often spiked with seal or dog penis or other exotica. It's too big a moral price to pay, and it's unnecessary. There are great, fortifying vegetarian aphrodisiac herbs.

One such pleasant tea is called Vitality Tea for Men, made by Butterfly Brand in San Francisco. It contains epimedium, a top-quality adrenal tonic that is a precursor of testosterone, combined with ligusticum, a blood-building herb that strongly increases circulation and a couple of other herbs that bring the improved circulation to the place in question. Drink a cup or two hot during the afternoon and evening for a feeling of sexual well-being.

# Recommended for Women

In American health food stores the female equivalents of male performance herbal combinations have names such as Woman's Treasure or Woman's Harmony, distributed by Health Concerns in Oakland. They contain mostly Chinese tonic herbs that regulate menstruation and treat PMS. Other useful herbal remedies are vitex, also called chaste berry, a popular herb in Europe, used to balance hormones. Change-O-Life and other such estrogenic herbal combinations were covered in Chapter 12 on menopause. The natural stimulation of estrogen with these herbal products will make you feel younger and more beautiful.

Although hormonal issues are related to sex, you may enjoy additional aphrodisiac herbs to enhance satisfaction. Among aphrodisiac herbs suitable for women, I prefer the following combination that builds both sexual fluids and strength. Unless you have dizziness, a headache or fever, you can use this healing tea to mend sexual weakness and fatigue.

## Fo-Ti Lift Tea

Take two capsules of the moistening herb fo-ti *(Polygonum multiflori)*, available in health food stores or from Chinatown shops, where it is called Shou Wu Pien. It also comes as a liquid extract, Shou Wu Chih, in which case you should use two tablespoons. At the same time drink a cup of hot clove-and-cinnamon tea, using one-quarter teaspoon clove powder, one-eighth teaspoon cinnamon powder, and one pinch of sea salt to a cup of hot water.

Drinking this brew, you will feel a warm, relaxing sensation as the energy circulation in your pelvic area opens. If you use this combination on a regular basis, your periods will become smoother and sex will not tire you.

## Emotional Upset

If you are depressed, anxious, or tired, you won't feel like making love. You first have to remove emotional and energy blocks. I like homeopathic remedies because they are safe, fast-acting, and easy to find. Just add a dose of homeopathic pills or extract to a little water or let them melt under your tongue and you will be able to let go of the day. Although these remedies work for both sexes, I imagine women will be more able to use them in teas to complement their cooking. This can be done in your healing space or anywhere as long as you wait twenty minutes after eating or drinking coffee before taking a homeopathic remedy.

You should use the remedies one at a time for long-term or acute upsets, depending on the homeopathic strength. Lower strengths such as 6x are commonly used five times daily for chronic problems or as often as every fifteen minutes for acute problems; or one or two doses of 30c is often enough for acute problems. Occasionally, a symptom may become slightly worse with the first dose of a remedy but will disappear with the second dose. All but homeopathic aconite can be used on a long-term basis. You can cancel the action of a homeopathic remedy at any time by drinking one cup of regular or decaffeinated coffee.

For depression, weeping, and thick sinus congestion, use homeopathic pulsatilla 30c.

For anxiety, panic, or fear, use homeopathic aconite 30c. Stop using the remedy when it makes you perspire slightly.

For worry, guilt, loss, and grief, use homeopathic ignatia 30c.

For fatigue from stress and severe diarrhea, use homeopathic arsenicum 30c.

## Fatigue—the Great Anaphrodisiac

An anaphrodisiac is something that takes away desire. Fatigue makes us feel vulnerable, abused, or closed. We may want to avoid sharing our feelings. The Fo-Ti Lift Tea recipe I invented is a strong energy stimulant suitable for either sex. The following herbs, available in Asian herb shops and health food stores, are very useful for sexual weakness and exhaustion. They treat chronic problems such as aching lower back and legs, frequent clear-colored urination, chills, frequent yawning, weak muscle strength, anxiety, and depression. Avoid taking them when you have a cold.

Ashwagandha is the East Indian equivalent of Chinese ginseng, although it is a stronger sexual tonic. It is not as warming as ginseng, but it cures backache from muscle strain. For that reason, it is also recommended for weak expectant mothers. Add one-half teaspoon to tea anytime, unless you have a fever or headache.

Sexoton is a pill found in Chinese herb shops that treats fatigue, asthma with wheezing, diarrhea, and urinary incontinence from low adrenal energy. It contains both blood-building and energy-tonic herbs. Use it when you're so tired you don't want to see anyone. The normal dosage is six to ten pills three times daily, but you will feel beneficial results faster by finding your individual dosage.

# A Deep-Acting Vitality Tea

The following light, delicate-tasting tea provides a source of rejuvenating energy and inspiration because it replenishes kidney and adrenal energy. Chinese medicine considers the water element to be the foundation of sexuality, hormone balance, strength, endurance, mental clarity, and good memory.

This tea may not solve all your problems but it can put you back on your feet after exhaustion from overwork, drugs, jet lag, or too many stimulants. The tea is not jet fuel—it may not increase your drive for achievement or sexual pleasure—but it will allow you to feel renewed, refreshed and revitalized.

Its ingredients are simple—a handful of leaves and berries. In China a similar brew is used to simulate the healing powers of deer antler, which rebuilds damaged bone marrow and bone strength. This tea is especially useful for anyone recovering from illness, fever, or wasting diseases as well as extreme chronic fatigue.

## *Letha's Deep-Rejuvenating Serum*

**1 handful of *Epimedium grandiflorum* (yin yang huo)**
**1 handful of *Fructus lychii* (gou ji tse)**

Simmer the herbs in 1 quart of spring water for twenty minutes and drink one cup of the warm tea at a time. The dosage is three or more cups daily. Separate the tea from meals so you can feel its full benefit. Do not use garlic or hot spices that day. The Deep-Rejuvenating Serum is not digestive because it actually works much deeper than digestive herbs and spices in order to renew your deepest reservoir of life force.

# A Hormonal Massage

Most people destroy their vitality with overwork, worry, and bad habits. This massage is an excellent way to rejuvenate while revitalizing your sexual hormones. It is not sexual in the usual sense because you do it with a loved one or alone but without having sex. That way you get the full benefit of boosting youth-giving hormones without paying the price of fatigue.

For lovers, this massage might be the crowning glory of a lovely evening. Or you might use it to harmonize energies with dear friends of either sex. It is a healing treatment aimed at preventing aging and also feelings of depression and isolation.

The massage is a reward. You may need to spend some months preparing for healthy sex by taking herbs such as gotu kola to settle your nerves or ashwagandha to build sexual strength. But this massage can be done by anyone, even people who are very weak. You might fix a delicious aphrodisiac meal, using ginger, clove, and garlic. Eat light, healthy foods. If you're alone for the evening, don't pass up this opportunity for personal well-being: Think of this massage as a daily fitness exercise for a younger, more beautiful you.

Do not practice this massage if you are angry, upset, or have a full stomach. Wait two hours after eating, and avoid hot or cold extremes in room temperature. Do not rush into this practice, expecting it to be perfect; take time to explore your experience. Excess talking spends energy and breath. Speak few words and then softly, with love.

## In Your Healing Space

After a hot bath, pat yourself dry with perfumed towels dabbed with sweet-pungent fragrance oils such as sage, clove, or rosemary. They open the senses. Warm your hands by rubbing them together with a few drops of raw sesame oil.

Sit facing each other, holding hands, and synchronize your breathing so that the same steady breath flows between you.

After a few moments, each person should place the right hand over the other's heart, while holding left hands. Close your eyes and continue breathing slowly and smoothly. When ready, continue your harmonious breathing while you massage each other. I like to give massage while listening to very slow East Indian music, but you can use music that inspires you.

Gently massage each other's ears, head, neck, shoulders, and collarbone. Using the tips of your fingers, massage from under the collarbone down the middle of the chest, making extra space between the ribs. Be gentle and spend extra time with painful areas to smooth away tension.

## For Women

Do this for yourself or have your partner do it: Seated in a comfortable position, gently and slowly massage each breast with circular motions counterclockwise fifty times. Use sesame oil, adding a drop of White Flower Oil or White Tiger Balm to stimulate deeper breathing. Or use a massage oil that contains lavender. Massage of the breast releases necessary female hormones that tone the uterus and female organs while deepening sensuality. During the breast massage, imagine a garden of fresh flowers in your uterus.

Lying down, apply a few drops of sesame or lavender oil to the lower abdomen and both sides of the groin. Warm the abdomen with about fifty slow clockwise circles, gathering energy into the navel. Then warm the groin gently with the palms of your hands. That opens the sexual area for better circulation. The ovaries are above the groin on either side of the pubic bone. Warming and gently massaging this area protects the health of the ovaries and is relaxing. Gently massaging the ovaries, inhale, lock the anus closed, and send your sexual energy up to your third eye.

Then press downward along the inside of the thighs and legs to release tension stored there. Continue massaging all the way down to the feet and rub the soles briskly with sesame oil. Put on clean cotton socks.

Press the lower back at the waist to release pressure and fatigue there. Or lie flat on a wooden back-roller and let it iron out your aching muscles. Your tired adrenal energy will feel improved.

## For Men

Do this for yourself or have your partner do it for you: Warm your hands by rubbing them together with a little sesame oil. After massaging the upper body as described above, apply a few drops of the oil to the lower abdomen and groin area. While lying down, warm the abdomen with fifty gentle clockwise movements, gathering energy into the navel. Warm the groin area with the palms of the hands and press gently to release the area.

Place the hands gently to warm the sexual organs. Using the soft part of your fingertips, massage with counterclockwise movements the area above and around the entire scrotum. This brings blood circulation to the area, increases testosterone, and helps prevent prostrate congestion. The sexual area will feel invigorated. Continue as long as it's comfortable. Then relax, inhale, lock the anus closed, and visualize your energy moving upward to your third eye. That recharges the pituitary gland, a master gland for rejuvenation.

When you are ready to continue, press the inner thighs to relax tense muscles and massage all the way down to the feet. Rub sesame oil into the soles of the feet.

Control the urge to have sex by stopping movement completely, breathing deeply, and lifting your energy out of the groin, up through the top of your head. That way you can benefit from the rejuvenating effects of increasing hormones and sexual vitality.

## Being Together with Love

Sit close, facing each other, heart to heart, with your hands warming each other's lower back at the waist. Continue breathing slowly as you form a complete energy circle. Send your awareness up through your body to your third eye and put your foreheads together. Imagine your collective energy rising up the front of you and down your backs in two intersecting circles. You might stay that way for a long time, perhaps hours, chanting prayers or quietly blended in ecstasy, feeling your love as a spiritual fountain you both share.

When you are alone, practice the same rejuvenating massage for yourself, but at the end, sit in a comfortable position or propped up with pillows. Imagine your favorite deity or highest inspiration to be your partner or witness.

## Keys

Pale tongue: Warming tonic herbs and foods—ginger, clove, fenugreek, ashwagandha.

Red tongue: Cooling, moistening herbs and foods—asparagus, cilantro, parsley, sarsaparilla, fo-ti (he shou wu herb, Shou Wu Pien pills)

Links: Also see Chapters 3 (diets), 7, 8 (winter), 9, 10, 12, 13

# CHAPTER 15

# Finding New Meaning in Work

*For those on the fast track.*

*Your Goals:* To do the best work you can and never get tired or bored, to improve your vitality and mental acuity while on the job, and to reduce stress, your worst addiction.

*Materials:* Nori seaweed for salt cravings. Fennel seeds, cinnamon sticks, healthy sugar substitutes, and Chyavanprash for sweet cravings. Antioxidants such as ginkgo and grape-seed extract; clove tea for wheezing asthma and shortness of breath; Raw Tienchi Ginseng powder for poor circulation, chest pains, high cholesterol, and bruising. Homeopathic aconite 30c for panic; homeopathic belladonna 30c for heatstroke, rage, and pounding headaches. Curing Pills, Xiao Yao Wan, or teas made from ginger, mint, and tarragon for indigestion, and powdered cinnamon and turmeric for poor circulation. East Indian Shilajit capsules or homeopathic carbo. veg. 30c (homeopathic charcoal) for weak digestion and puffy abdomen. Homeopathic nux. vomica 30c for hangovers. Gotu kola capsules for improving memory and concentration. Valerian capsules for migraines, dizziness, and jet lag. Lots of green tea and green tea capsules for energy, vitality, mental focus, and prevention of illness.

When personal renewal extends into every corner of our life, it presents new insights that destroy a dull work routine. Vitality fuels confidence and humor. Herbs may not be able to make you compassionate, courageous, brilliant, or cheerful, but they can help you get past the tough spots. A bit of extra energy can make the difference between a job well done and being done in. This chapter is a bridge between Part Four and Part Five, providing herbal help for people who aim for the top and over-the-top of their profession.

I've met eighty-year-olds who were full of youthful drive and spunk. They live passionately and thrive. I have friends who burn a groove in their road to success. Using the wisdom of herbs, they stay physically and mentally fit. Successful people do more than deal with stress: they chase after it. A large part of success may be self-image, but most of it requires energy to keep up with or bound over the fast track.

# Break Through the Age Barrier

What kind of work can you see yourself doing in ten or twenty years? How do you want to involve yourself with people? Imagine yourself in an ideal work situation. What skills do you have to learn? It's wise to seek personal models of beautiful, productive, mature people. Have you ever watched an older person and thought, "I want to be like that when I'm older. I like that person's energy"?

# In Your Healing Space

Imagine the older person you want to become. Aim for age one hundred. The statistics are with you. People are living longer and better than ever. Wise people welcome every opportunity to grow, to begin something new. Some of my friends can serve as examples to help you. I offer a survey of their health routines, especially the ways they deal with stress and aging at work.

# Life in High Gear

Mieko, the senior Japanese female executive official and one of the most respected women at the United Nations, is in charge of policy coordination of African development and Asia-Africa cooperation. Recently she led a mission composed of representatives of several Asian nations, including Japan and China, to Ghana to establish a manufacturing operation capable of producing some nine hundred traditional herbal formulas. About 80 percent of Ghanaians regularly use herbal medicines.

Mieko is beautiful, sleek, and young-looking with a smile that makes everyone happy. She is highly creative and bold. She says her job demands "confidence, courage, strength, and faith in what you want to do." Her mother, nearly eighty and living in Japan, wanted to be a pilot. Encouraging Mieko to achieve all that a man could, she sent her "out into the world to become international."

Natural herbal medicines are very popular in Japan. Mieko says that herbs play a part in Japanese people's daily lives. That's interesting when you consider that on average Japanese people live at least ten years longer than Americans. (See Intelligent Choice, an excellent source of Japanese health products, in the Herbal Access section.)

## Seaweeds

For her everyday well-being, Mieko enjoys seaweeds. Every other day she eats nori, which is high in protein. Other favorites are kombu and wakame, which she adds to soups. Mieko feels that seaweed is important for women's menstrual health. It is high in minerals, especially potassium and iodine, which is essential for hormone balance. Mieko's high-energy diet of fish, rice, cleansing sour foods such as pickled vegetables, and phytoestrogenic soy products, including miso and tofu, keep her beautiful. She also likes to eat leeks or scallions, which are blood-cleansers, daily.

## A Good Hot Soak

Jet lag is endemic to Mieko's profession because she travels one-third of the year in Africa, Asia, and Europe. Her favorite cure for jet lag is a long, extremely hot bath. She always adds some of the refreshing lemon- or jasmine-scented Japanese bath crystals made by Osen or Tsumura, available from Yaohan in Los Angeles. (See the Herbal Access section for these and other Japanese health and beauty remedies.)

# Mental Focus

Another powerful woman is Eileen Heckart, star of stage, screen, and television, now in her seventies. Her home in Connecticut is filled with acting mementos including an Oscar she won in 1972 for her performance in *Butterflies Are Free*. Eileen's style is direct and earnest. Her Irish wit and high energy level are job requirements. As a stage actress, she says, "Every part requires background. You have to be a different person with every role." For example, Eileen read over thirty books before she played Eleanor Roosevelt. On stage, Eileen becomes someone else. She can forget her discomforts. It's part of her professionalism.

## Antioxidants

Eileen depends on sensitivity, intuition, and memory for her work. To keep herself primed for action, she protects her mental acuity with antioxidants. She takes a daily regime of Omega 3 fish oils, vitamins C and E, and minerals, including folic acid, potassium, magnesium, and selenium. She also takes acidophilus for her digestion. Her daily herbs include Ginkgold capsules, each 40 mg of ginkgo leaf, made by Nature's Way. Ginkgo, an antioxidant, protects memory and alertness by increasing blood circulation to the brain.

Eileen uses Nine Ginsengs, made by the same company. Most forms of ginseng are adaptogens, which means they help overcome stress by increasing endurance and regulating body temperature.

## The Power of Breath

Breathing is always a problem for smokers like Eileen. Reduced oxygen from damaged lungs leads to low energy. A doctor once told Eileen that

# Major Rejuvenation Herbs

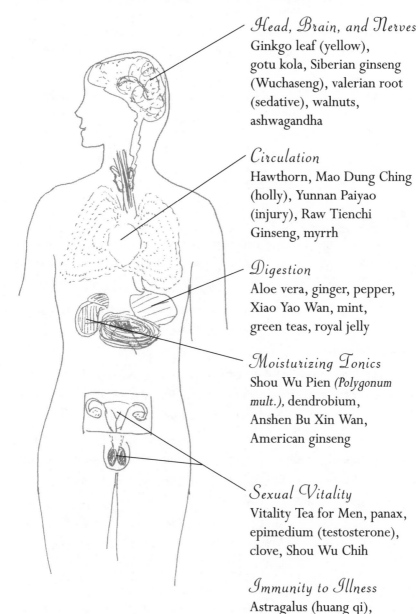

### Head, Brain, and Nerves
Ginkgo leaf (yellow),
gotu kola, Siberian ginseng
(Wuchaseng), valerian root
(sedative), walnuts,
ashwagandha

### Circulation
Hawthorn, Mao Dung Ching
(holly), Yunnan Paiyao
(injury), Raw Tienchi
Ginseng, myrrh

### Digestion
Aloe vera, ginger, pepper,
Xiao Yao Wan, mint,
green teas, royal jelly

### Moisturizing Tonics
Shou Wu Pien *(Polygonum
mult.)*, dendrobium,
Anshen Bu Xin Wan,
American ginseng

### Sexual Vitality
Vitality Tea for Men, panax,
epimedium (testosterone),
clove, Shou Wu Chih

### Immunity to Illness
Astragalus (huang qi),
Rheishi mushroom (ling zhi)

her voice lessons have helped her because she knows how to breathe properly and project her voice. Ping Chuan Wan, Chinese herbal pills for emphysema, have also helped her endurance.

One of Eileen's sons, Luke Yankee, is charm on wheels. He began acting in *Oliver* on stage at age seven. Now a director, he has worked with stars like Dick Clark, Rex Harrison, and Quincy Jones, from New York's Radio City Music Hall to Hollywood's Ovation Awards. Handsome, blond, over six feet tall, he occasionally strikes people as a young Laurence Olivier.

## Protection from Burnout

When Luke consulted me in New York for an herbal energy boost and complained about his sweet tooth, I recommended Chyavanprash, a healthy chocolate substitute found in East Indian groceries. (See page 112.) Vrrooom Power, pills distributed by Health Concerns of Oakland, California, works well for people who react to stress by reaching for sugar, sweets, salty foods, and hot spices. It helps normalize blood sugar and rebuild the baseline energy harmed by those stimulants.

Today Luke's apartment overlooks the famous Hollywood sign. He has no health complaints, thanks to a love match that was the "greatest thing that ever happened" to him. However, to prevent Hollywood director-producer burnout, I have recommended that he take one teaspoon of Raw Tienchi Ginseng powder in juice morning and evening. This anti-inflammatory herb encourages healthy blood circulation and reduces cholesterol, chest pain, internal bleeding, and bruises. Raw tienchi is appropriate for hot and fast people who are always thirsty or who are dehydrated from jet lag, late nights, or chronic fever conditions. Such cooling tonics are also ideal for hot flashes, hypertension, and diabetes.

Cooling blood tonic herbs increase body fluids to moisten internal organs and improve the appearance of skin and hair. Two moistening tonics for beautiful skin can be made into a mild-tasting tea by simmering a handful each of American ginseng and dendrobium in a quart of spring water for twenty minutes. Unfortunately, most of my meetings with Luke are now at airport restaurants, where he is between flights that take him around the world to direct new plays or television.

# The Will to Create

Ursule Molinaro is queenly, poised somewhere between this century and the ancient Greeks she writes about. I've been in awe of her ever since we met over thirty years ago. As a kid growing up in France, she had participated in the underground and had survived capture and torture by the Nazis.

Ursule always wears black, down to her black nail polish. I never thought of it as a sign of negativity or depression. Ursule is the essential female, the yin principle. Black for her is the artistic void into which spirits enter. With them, she fills her canvases, books, and imagination. She is a dragon lady, tiny and birdlike, with monstrous creative energy.

Her marble tabletop is usually strewn with artistic clutter—notes for a book she's writing, a dish of almonds, a few bottles of homeopathic tissue salts, and a half-empty wineglass. Her paintings of cats, deer, bears, and women in fancy hats charge her apartment with a lively softness.

## Blood Building and Centering

Over the years, Ursule has kept herself well with homeopathic minerals such as ferrum phosphate (iron) for feverish conditions or pain, calcium fluoride for weakness and poor circulation, and potassium phosphate for nervous conditions. More recently she has relied on a combination of vitamins, trace minerals, and amino acids called Personal Radical Shield, made by Smart Basics in San Francisco. Among the Chinese herbs I have recommended for her, Ursule prefers several pill remedies.

Liu Wei Di Huang Wan, also called Six Flavor Tea, is used to reverse dry cough, thirst, dry skin, blood deficiency, stiff lower back, muscle spasms, afternoon fevers, night sweats, and weakness from blood loss. I recommend two or three handfuls of the small pills daily for people who are dehydrated from smoking or overwork. A moistening tonic such as this should be avoided during colds and flu or chills with runny mucus.

Another Chinese remedy Ursule favors is called Curing Pills. Used to prevent and treat diarrhea, nausea, car sickness, and generally weak digestion with abdominal pain, it is very centering. It can also be used for the early stages of the common cold. Each small red box is one dose to be taken after or instead of meals. I find that the weakening effects of allergy season are reduced with one dose of Curing Pills.

Dan Shen Wan is a combination of camphor and Chinese red sage, which smooths and strengthens heart action while it reduces cholesterol. If you have thick ankles from water retention, a weak heart, chest pains, or high cholesterol, take four Dan Shen Wan pills daily after meals and reduce dietary fats and sweets.

*Using herbs, you come to know yourself by observing your energy.*

# The Joy of Being a Child at Play

Jean Claude van Itallie is a sprite. His eyes are blue crystal balls. He almost glitters with vitality. With a deliciously musical laugh, he's a human tuning fork who catches your energy and spins it back to you. He personifies living theater.

Jean Claude, one of the original La Mama playwrights, has written over thirty original plays and translations as well as widely produced English versions of Chekhov's major plays. In the 1960s he was the principle playwright for the Open Theater. One of his best-known plays is based on the *Tibetan Book of the Dead*. Traditionally, Buddhist monks chanted prayers during the time of a person's dying in order to safely guide the spirit to its next lifetime. Jean Claude's play has been widely performed and adapted as an opera. North Atlantic Books recently published his illustrated book, *The Tibetan Book of the Dead for Reading Aloud*.

He feels that to be a good playwright, you have to be a good actor and vice versa. To become an actor you must develop body, speech, and mind. For him, acting is a means to enlightenment. He says, "I don't like to teach just playwriting. I like to teach everything I do—writing, teaching, performing, meditating, everything—all rolled together. Counterculture . . . I'm not anti-mind. I just don't like the head detached from the body." Applause Books in New York has recently published Jean Claude's *The Playwright's Workbook.*

I've visited him in his New York pied-à-terre, an airy Japanese-style floating cloud, and also in his large monasterylike home in Rowe, Massachusetts. In 1977 it became the court for Trungpa Rinpoche, a tulku and leader of Kagyu Tibetan Buddhists.

## Balancing the Elements

An actor-activist, Jean Claude has worked for years with local political action groups to shut down nuclear power plants in his New England area. His high energy and clarity of purpose are enhanced by his health habits. For seventeen years he closely followed a vegan diet of fruits, vegetables, and a few grains. Such a diet provides boundless energy and enthusiasm as it clears the aura of meat, chemicals, and sludge, but it can weaken people who require a grounding, warming diet. It can leave a person spacey, thin, dehydrated, and undersexed if it fails to nourish internal organs.

People who follow vegan or raw food diets need to combine proteins and minerals carefully, using digestive herbs and spices when necessary in order to ensure adequate absorption. Tofu, seaweeds, and grain combinations such as corn and beans are complete proteins. Mineral-rich herbs, especially nettles, alfalfa, and spirolina supply energy and build immunity to infections and allergies. Bay leaf tea settles the stomach very well for people who eat primarily raw food diets.

Jean Claude's teacher, Trungpa, was concerned that his diet was extreme for a different reason. Asian doctor-philosophers believe that people balance one type of energy with its opposite. If we feel feverish or overheated, we can eat cooling foods and herbs. Balancing energy goes even further. Spiritual leaders aim to improve our thinking. Even the best-intentioned spiritual practices, when left unchecked by questioning, can end up waving the flag of ego. To challenge Jean Claude's ironclad diet, Trungpa ordered him to eat a steak. Jean Claude learned that he is more than what he eats. At the same time, he felt comfortable and grounded from the meat. There had to be another way.

## An East Indian Rejuvenating Herb

I recommended that Jean Claude take Shilajit, an Ayurvedic medicine in capsule form available in East Indian groceries. It is actually bitumen, a processed form of coal, used to rebuild sexual fluids as it rids the body of impurities. Ayurveda classifies Shilajit as a major rejuvenating tonic that rebuilds resistance to fatigue and stress. I also told Jean Claude about my deep-rejuvenating serum (page 231), which he enjoys drinking in the evening.

# New Beginnings

I can't remember how and when I first met Salima. She has always been a ray of sunlight for me. She calls her friends precious because they are a gift from God. *Salima* is the Arabic word for "peace of God," and Salima is a minister in her own church of love. A beautiful black woman, she was born Ira Swain in Kansas, and became an opera singer and voice teacher. When she reached spiritual maturity, she took the name of her Sufi sheik, Muhaiyaddeen, so that now she is called Salima Muhaiyaddeen.

Together with fifty close friends, I attended her naming ceremony, where we sang together and talked about our love of life. Salima repeated the Arabic names of God like a prayer of hope. She looked radiant in long African robes. Earlier that year, at age fifty, she had completed her first New York Marathon after running for seven hours.

In addition to performing in classical and spiritual music concerts, Salima teaches music therapy in New York to children with speech problems and voice to adults who want to grow spiritually. The healing power of music has kept her and her voice students happy and well. She begins with breathing exercises to build strength and courage. She uses therapeutic touch to free blocked areas of the body. Her work always includes music with a positive, healing message.

In December 1997, with fifty Sufi friends from Philadelphia, Salima made a pilgrimage called Umra to Mecca to reaffirm her faith. In her

words, she connected with the person she wanted to grow into. To keep
her energy clear and vital, she eats dandelion greens and takes capsules.
Her voice is kept strong with the antimucus foods she eats daily—fresh
ginger used in cooking and clove and basil tea.

# The Ever New, Ever Open Mind

Kati and Desi Bognar, Hungarian-American friends of ours in Peacham,
Vermont, fixed a smashing Nigerian curry one summer evening. World
travelers both, Desi has written books on filmmaking and a guide to
famous Hungarians. Kati has lectured on the joys and health benefits of
Hungarian cooking. That evening they introduced us to Bill Lederer,
author of The Ugly American.

Fate placed that book in my hands when I was ten. From about the age
of seven on, I had a great interest in all things Oriental. I admired Chinese
porcelains, Japanese paintings of misty landscapes, and pentatonic music.
I studied maps of Asia and decided where I wanted to visit. The Ugly
American was one of the first doors I walked through to get there.

## Freedom in Movement

Bill is tall, slim, and straight as a pine. At eighty-seven he wants to return
to Szechuan for a bicycle trip. Recently he moved from Vermont to Florida
to live "on a small pond with many cranes, cormorants, and seabirds." He
explains, "I am a person who requires much exercise. Being able to swim
every day either in a wonderful pool or in the ocean nourishes me."

Full of stories about his life in China in the 1940s when he was
assigned by the U.S. Navy to tail Chou En-lai, Bill reminds me of two
other long-lived writers who were military intelligence men—Lawrence
Durrell and John Blofeld. Bill's stories have an ironic twist. Some end in
a joke on himself. With blunt candor, he has a journalist's quick grasp of
people. His mind, constantly at work composing stories, keeps him young.

Bill gets up at 5:00 A.M. and drinks his morning glass of apple juice
and hot coffee. He fasts on vegetable broth in a Swiss spa for a couple of

weeks each year. He also does a form of yoga he learned at a temple in Thailand. Watching him speak, I noticed how at home Bill is in his body. He describes how James Michener wrote six hours a day until he died at age ninety, and how Robert Frost walked stooping forward, swinging his arms. Bill gets up to demonstrate.

## The Importance of Kindness

That evening at dinner, Bill told a story of how Ernest Hemingway had taught him about kindness. Bill, a young navy ensign, had won a case of Scotch while gambling. In China, under heavy Japanese bombing in the 1940s, everyone, including the top military brass, tried to buy his Scotch, but Bill wouldn't sell a drop. Hemingway flashed a huge roll of hundred-dollar bills. Bill told the famous older writer that he would trade three bottles for six writing lessons. Hemingway took the Scotch and gave Bill only five lessons.

When Hemingway was about to leave on a military boat, Bill reminded him of the last lesson. Hemingway looked him in the eye and said, "This is the most important lesson you will ever learn: that Scotch was tea, but I didn't tell anyone because you would have been laughed off this base as a fool. People are a miserable lot and writers are worse than most. But to be a great writer, you have to learn compassion."

That is a lesson I am still learning. Bill is a wry gentleman with a keen sense of observation and dedication to seeking knowledge who is kept young by his work. Meeting him fills me with a spark charged with exciting possibilities: I feel that I am only half finished with my life.

## A Passionate Life

If I could shape my life's work after any one person, it would be Dr. Bernard Jensen. He has been a courageous seeker of wisdom and leader of the American natural health movement for nearly seventy years. Today, at age ninety, still teaching health seminars around the country, he radiates the generosity of a highly attuned spirit. America's leading holistic nutritionist, he has devoted his life to the search for, study, and use of whole, pure, natural, and fresh foods in building health, happiness, and longevity.

The practical health information found in his nearly sixty books is based on the at-times amazing success stories of the more than 350,000 people he has helped in his clinics. He has also traveled to remote areas—including China, Tibet, and the Hunza Valley, where he found people living well past the age of one hundred—to search out the best natural cures and foods for enhanced intelligence and longevity.

Bernard Jensen's personal vitality has been a well-deserved reward for his studies. As a young student at West Coast Chiropractic College he abused his health with junk foods. After graduation he collapsed and was diagnosed with an incurable lung disease. Refusing to accept the diagnosis, he sought the advice of a Seventh-Day Adventist doctor who taught him basic nutritional principles. He began to eat a safe, clean diet with many colors and high vibrations made up of fruits, vegetables, seeds, grains—all natural, organic vegetarian foods.

Using his own nutritional methods, he was able to cure his prostate cancer in the mid-1990s. Soon after tests showed the cancer was under control, he and his wife were in an automobile accident that left him paralyzed from the hips down. Again, he pulled through the agony and apparent hopelessness of his situation with courage, determination, and special nutritional support. Mrs. Jensen says that he fasted for four months on carrot juice and water "to clear out everything that shouldn't be there." Then he drank milk fresh from a goat. Today he walks fine without a cane.

Bernard Jensen has received many international awards, gold medals, and honorary degrees for his work in health and for his humanitarian service from institutions such as the Academy of Science in Paris, the Center for the Study of Human Sciences in Lisbon, the World Congress of Scientific Medicine in Italy, and the International Naturopathic Association. He was knighted into the Order of St. John of Malta in 1978. In 1982, Dr. and Mrs. Jensen traveled to Brussels to accept the Dag Hammarskjold Award of the Pax Mundi Academy for his exceptional service to humanity. At the age of 75, he received his Ph.D. in clinical nutrition from the University of Humanistic Studies in San Diego.

He retired from active practice in 1983 to his ranch in Escondido, where he devotes himself to teaching, writing, and lecturing on nutrition, rejuvenation, and iridology, an effective form of diagnosis.

Modern medicine makes a strong case for genes and germs in determining our health. Bernard Jensen has said that he was born out of a Danish pastry. His mother died at age thirty of consumption. His healing methods do not rely on laboratory animal testing, drugs, or a "smile for the surgeon" attitude. Jensen returns to the kitchen. Using natural, pure foods, sunshine, fresh air, exercise, and a wise spirit, he has made himself over from scratch for the purpose of helping humanity.

# The Path of Adventure

Alexandra David-Neel was also an inspiration for me. She became famous for walking directly into the eye of a storm. In 1924, against direct orders from the British Empire, despite war, plague, bandits, freezing temperatures, and her own poor sense of direction, she navigated her way from Sikkim to Lhasa, Tibet, with a pocket compass, getting lost only once or twice. Disguised as a beggar, she and her adopted son, a Tibetan tulku (an evolved spirit), traveled alone because the journey was forbidden. They proved that knowledge cannot be kept secret or owned by a privileged class.

Alexandra David-Neel's health habits were not prudent, especially on long trips. She would fast while trekking, then feast when she rested. A petite woman, in later years she ballooned to a weight of nearly two hundred pounds. One good habit that she maintained, however—a trust of homeopathic remedies—came from her French background. To boost energy and mental clarity during exhaustion, she took homeopathic strychnine. Trouble arose if she took too much or was too weak: she temporarily got lost. She hardly looked at maps but relied on instinct and the advice of other pilgrim travelers.

A safe homeopathic energy booster is homeopathic arsenicum 30c. It treats physical collapse and diarrhea from weakness. I never met Alexandra

David-Neel, who died in 1968 at age 101, but through her letters and her biography, *The Secret Lives of Alexandra David-Neel* (Overlook Press, 1998), I feel I have traveled with her.

## Courage and Karma

Michael Foster, David-Neel's biographer, respects the "rational-mystical" form of Buddhism. Like the hermits who practiced secret rites in caves and respected the Buddha of pure truth, the test-all-authority Buddha known to those familiar with Gautama's original works, Michael believes that the essential human virtue is not piety but courage. His fate has led him from childhood Brooklyn street fights to writing best-sellers. His mightiest sword is an evolved spirit.

As a young man, he quit a full scholarship program at Harvard Law School to join Che Guevara in Latin America. He never found Che in the confusion of war but wrote historical novels and biographies instead. Those who have an ability to discard personal safety and success while losing themselves in the process of creation are most alive. Those who can thus create and remain generous and loving are enlightened. Michael has a sweet, generous disposition, but is obsessive about work. He can lose his temper. Like Trungpa, he holds dear a "Be here now" approach to life and work. He writes neither for acclaim nor for personal success, generously sharing the spotlight with his wife, who sometimes helps him with research. He is a perfectionist because he feels that he must use his extraordinary talent for the common good.

Michael always works on several books at once. Fatigue has raised his blood pressure, but he finds quick relief from dizziness, headaches, and hot temper with two Chinese herbal remedies, Blood Pressure Repressing Tablets and Antihypertensive Tea.

## Sugar, Hours of Sitting, and Gout

You don't have to be a writer to develop gout, a particularly painful form of arthritis that usually attacks the fingers and toes. Writing books does not bring on the pain, but sitting long hours without moving, while eating acidic foods for energy, will. Is your big toe swollen, hot, and throbbing? You too may have gout.

Belladonna, a deadly plant found in nature, when prepared in homeopathic form, can eliminate headaches and hot, sharp pains and redness in joints. Add one dose of homeopathic belladonna 30c to a glass of water and sip it throughout the day for gout or for burning, throbbing pain, fevers, or ear infections. Other homeopathic remedies especially useful for gout are homeopathic sodium phosphate (nat. phos. 6x), which eliminates acid and homeopathic formica rufa 6x (homeopathic ant), which is diuretic.

## The Nexus of the Plexus

From our point of view, all the people in this chapter have something in common: to varying degrees, they deny their health to give full range to their work. This may sound like an Eastern road to enlightenment, but torturing the body can actually lead to mental dullness, fatigue, poor hearing, and weak memory. The people I have described are outstanding because they manage to be productive despite the demands of their work or their bad habits. They are rare. Most of us who sit at a desk all day need the same kind of herbal help that great writers, diplomats, and performers do. We do our best work when we feel comfortable and centered.

# Digestive Remedies and Mental Clarity

Digesting ideas all day is rough work. It tends to wear out vitality and cause cramps. For anyone who has to sit or stand for long hours, I recommend herbs that free circulation, especially in the digestive center. Among the best digestive remedies are:

> Ginger, tarragon, and mint tea
>
> All forms of green or oolong tea and peppermint

Raw radishes and barley soup

Bee pollen and royal jelly

Acidophilus

Xiao Yao Wan (indigestion, hypoglycemia)

Curing Pills (nausea, diarrhea, and chills)

Bu Zhong Yi Qi Won (chronic diarrhea and weakness)

Sexoton is a Chinese patent remedy for tired, aching lower back, low energy, shortness of breath, diarrhea, and sexual weakness. Such an energy tonic cannot cure but can sometimes improve health after the attack on vitality that comes from drinking coffee. If you are overheated or have hypertension or diabetes, this remedy is too heating for you. It is better to use Liu Wei Di Huang Wan for inflammatory problems, including tight spasms in the lower back, night fevers and sweats, and thirst.

# Dealing with Addictions

The worst addiction is stress itself. If we didn't create the *habit* of fatigue, anxiety, and overwork, would we be so willing to continue it? Some people thrive on stress because they are bored with normality. Some get so used to stress that they flog themselves with addictions to maintain it. If you use caffeine, sweets, or alcohol to keep working, here are a few suggestions for how to drop a crutch before it turns into a club to beat yourself with. Chapter 17 will also help bring your cravings and need for stress into balance.

## Alcohol

Homeopathic nux vomica will strengthen the "no" response to excess rich food and alcohol. It is recommended for hangovers, bad temper, and indigestion resulting from overeating and drinking. The best way to reduce cloudy thinking and pain from a hangover is to take one dose of homeopathic nux vomica 30c after overeating or drinking. For preventing alcohol craving, during five consecutive days, take one dose of 200x nux vomica before bed and another one-half hour after meals. Then stop for one day and resume as needed. Avoid coffee while using this or any homeopathic remedy, or wait twenty minutes after drinking regular or decaffeinated coffee. Follow a healthy, simple diet such as the one found in Chapter 9 in order to cleanse the body and eliminate the irritating side effects of alcohol and stimulants. If you get a pounding, hot withdrawal headache, take a dose of homeopathic belladonna 30c.

## Cigarettes

I have heard people say that cigarettes give them a smoke screen to hide behind. Others say that smoking sharpens their wits. If you are tired of coughing behind your smoke screen, stop giving yourself and the people around you cancer. Quitting smoking will add years to your life, improve your skin, and, according to recent research, improve your memory almost immediately.

During my health practice, I have found that ear acupuncture worked quite well for curbing the physical addiction, although some people turned to other nervous habits. It is best to combine any stop-smoking treatment with a stress-reduction plan that includes nerve remedies such as eight to ten capsules daily of gotu kola, which heals the brain, or daily doses of homeopathic aconite 30c, used to stop panic and sudden headache.

At home, massage your ears front and back with a little sunflower or olive oil and then wash them. You will notice painful spots on your ears. Those point to areas in your body where inflammation has caused damage. Some parts of the ear may have red dots or blemishes. A drop of essential sandalwood oil or sunflower oil placed there with a Q-Tip will feel relaxing.

# You Are Unique and Remarkable

A whole world of experience opens up when you start planning for a long, productive future. No matter what your age, imagine reaching one hundred. You can't know for certain what you will need then, but you can visualize a full and satisfied life. Do not let your view be limited by your present circumstances, which can change in an eye blink. Natural remedies promote well-being because they connect you with the spirit and energy of eternal life. Some plants such as spirolina and ginkgo trees have been here since the dinosaurs. They are charged with the juices of creation. The first fruits of a new planet, they can fill you with life.

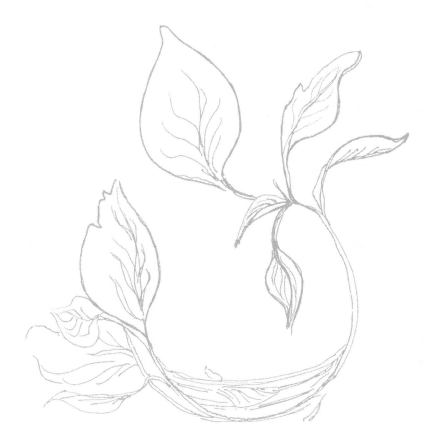

# PART FIVE

# LONGEVITY AND SPIRIT

*The aim of longevity is spirit,
and the method of spirit is love.*

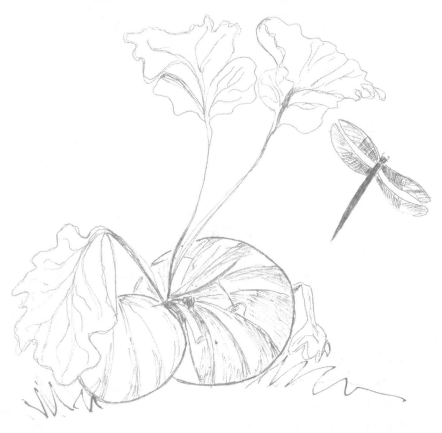

# Psychic Fire and the Roots
# of Chronic Illness and Injury

Now that you have learned skills for recovery from injury and illness, it's time to look deeper and address their hidden meaning. Contrary to popular scientific belief, not all illnesses occur because of genes or germs. You may also have developed some harmful living patterns. Try the following visualizations to find out what they are. If you consistently use the information in this part of the book, you will need to make fewer brilliant comebacks over the years.

## In Your Healing Space

Use your healing space as a sanctuary, where you feel protected enough to express any desire to yourself. Only you can grasp how it feels to be happy and whole. With the following visualization exercises, you will re-create the feeling of wellness you had before your problem occurred. If necessary, you will reach back to a former lifetime to feel the joy of health and youth.

People leave clues around the house, reminding them of their original self. You may have an old picture of yourself or someone else hidden in a drawer. It recalls a time and place where you felt protected, hopeful, or victorious. It occurred before your illness or unhappiness existed. Find that picture or memento now and place it in your healing space.

Visualize yourself back in that picture, or in your memory travel back to that time and place. Notice who is near you. Let those people, living or dead, be your companions now as you sit in your healing space. People you have loved and respected will always be a part of your life. Ask them for help now.

# Destroy the Negative

Illness and sadness are like evil spirits that get in the way of our progress. We will now dissolve them with the help of your protector companions. First, you have to clarify your impression of who or what is actually hurting you. Your illness or bad experience may be only a part of the problem. Sometimes even a happy event such as childbirth can lead to readjustments. The following mental exercise will help you sort things out for yourself.

Lying flat on your back in your healing space, place your hands over your navel and breathe deeply into your lower abdomen. Imagine your protector companions sitting around you.

Slowly visualize yourself ten years ago, remembering details about how you looked, what you were doing, and who you lived with. Mentally re-create that time and place in detail as you breathe deeply.

Then visualize yourself twenty years ago in the same way. Taking plenty of time, continue remembering back in detail ten years at a time until you reach childhood. Where were you at fifty, forty, thirty, twenty, and so on? Who was in your family? Who were your friends?

At some point in your visualization, you will start to breathe deeper and in a more relaxed manner. You will sense that your memory has opened up and taken you far back. It may be before this lifetime. That is the time we are aiming for. That is your period of balance and harmony. If you cannot sense that time of inner harmony, mentally complete these statements.

I was happy and positive until I met _____.
I was healthy until I _____.
My trouble started when _____.
I was fine until _____.

Now we will go back with your mind and destroy the trouble you have had since then—the who, when, and where that you filled the blanks with. Name them as the cause of your grief or imbalance. Calling their names is not strong enough to make them disappear. For that, we have to build a psychic fire.

# A Psychic Fire

Illness and depression can keep you from becoming your higher self. You have to be ruthless when destroying them. Call it magic or the power of creative thinking—you can purge yourself of those demons. Professional athletes, actors, and business executives have learned to overcome personal blocks in this way. By eliminating what is negative about your past, you can make room for new growth and joyful experience. In your effort to create psychic space, you may have to temporarily eliminate good memories about people and places to get at the poison. Don't worry—our visualization will eventually put everything in order.

Comfortably sitting in your healing space, light a candle on a table or on the floor in front of you. Visualize it as a huge fire capable of burning down tall buildings. Take time to breathe deeply, making the flame grow larger and brighter.

Count backward, starting from your present age and going to the year of your birth. As you remember each year, mentally put your personal demons into the fire until they are turned to cinders. Call them by name or burn pictures of them if it helps. Also realize that it is your hatred, disappointment, and grief over them that are hurting you. You must incinerate those feelings in the fire.

This exercise is more powerful than you know. Visualizations similar to this have been used by Tibetan monks trapped by snow in high passes. The psychic fire of meditation made them feel warm enough to dry wet sheets placed around them. It was more than a show of mental energy. Visualizations such as this become powerful when a spiritual component is added.

As you burn them up, send your enemies to another place. Invite them to leave, breaking all ties with you. You have already learned enough from your association with them, even though you may not be ready to forgive them. That can happen as you become stronger and wiser by using herbs.

# CHAPTER 16

# Heal Your
# Broken Heart

*Unleash your vitality
and find freedom to change.*

---

*Your Goal:* To look at grief in a different way; to free your stuck energy and trapped mind.

*Materials:* Homeopathic gelsemium 30c for anxiety about the future; homeopathic pulsatilla 30c for grief; homeopathic kali. sulph. 6x and ferrum phos. 6x to build immune strength. Holly, the Bach Flower remedy, for hatred. Ding Xin Wan or Siberian ginseng combined with gotu kola for better sleep; Xiao Yao Wan, Bu Zhong Yi Qi Wan, Saint John's wort, pure essential lavender oil, or rosebud tea for depression. Astragalus root for vitality and immunity to chronic weakness and fatigue-related illness, including cancer. Yunnan Paiyao or homeopathic arnica 30c for physical and psychological trauma.

---

In Burma, Aung San Suu Kyi, a wife and mother and the leader of the people's movement for democracy, sat locked up in a prison cell, unable to communicate with the world. Outside, thousands of her followers, her adopted children, were being killed. The suffering of so many was incomprehensible. The only weapon the Burmese mother of two, the daughter of one of the country's founders, had to fight against a corrupt, ruthless, authoritarian regime was her courage and determination—her heart. Her love for her country was returned by her people. Besides political prisoners trapped in cells, many more are trapped by their own hearts and minds.

Perhaps you are grieving for a love that ended too soon or one that never happened. This chapter will show you ways to regain emotional balance and build confidence. Some people say that we must derive benefit from suffering. Suffering has its limits. It's exhausting. Exhaustion clouds our perception. When pain becomes a means to self-understanding and self-expression, it becomes healing pain. Longing is the netherworld from which artistic creation springs, the sacred space before completion and wholeness, from where the soul reaches beyond itself. If you are longing for a loved one or filled with a sense of failure or rejection, you are beginning the art of becoming a new person. Your loss can become your best friend.

I clearly remember the first time I ever swore aloud. It was remarkable because I was brought up in a refined, artistic home where we hardly ever raised our voices. My soon-to-become ex-husband and I were having our last supper. I wore black. Having lived as students abroad and worked for ten years to pay for his expensive Ph.D., I had nothing—no career, no children, no home, not even a steady job. I seriously wanted a life. Later I heard that he had secretly stashed money aside during our troubled years together. I was down in the dumps financially, yet my attitude was positive. He told me that since I was thirty, I was *middle-aged* and that I would have to go downhill without him. I looked him square in the eye and let him have it.

Healing anger may have helped me through that first year alone, but it too has its limits. Anger is a knot in the stomach and a lump in the throat. It was ultimately love that helped me most. I would never have found that love if I hadn't been free to look for it. I soon changed everything about my life. Sometimes all you need is a tragedy to get you out of a comfortable trap.

The herbs we will use in this chapter heal heartache by freeing stuck circulation. When depressed, enraged, or grieving, you turn into a knot of tangled energy. A sudden shock or terrible news can make you feel a tightness or pain in the chest. That pain is the result of poor circulation, leading to inadequate oxygen flow. Easing chest pains may not eliminate the cause of your heartache, but it can increase the quantity of oxygen that reaches your brain. That will help you deal with your problems with a clearer head and more tranquil emotions. The problem may still be there, but you will be better able to handle it.

Once a woman described how her Chinese doctor saved her from surgery. Her Western doctor strongly suspected cancer when he found she had fibroids. One month before her scheduled surgery, the woman consulted a Chinese doctor who specialized in Qi Gong, a meditative form of movement and breathing aimed at building strength and endurance.

He advised her among other things to awaken and breathe deeply and calmly at 4:00 A.M. because the air in New York is cleaner at that time. That is also the time of day when our Qi energy rises to create immunity to illness. That practice had been part of the healing routine the Chinese doctor had used to cure himself of tuberculosis many years before.

I would have advised the woman to take alternating doses of homeopathic kali. sulph. 6x and ferrum phos. 6x (potassium and iron) all day— every hour on the hour—instead of rising at 4:00 A.M. But the Chinese doctor and I agree on the rest of her routine. He gave the woman Chinese medicinal herbs to help dissolve the fibroids.

After one month, following this health routine—to the amazement of her Western doctors—the fibroids had become much smaller. They were re-diagnosed as benign and removed. The woman had gained a great deal of strength, confidence, and emotional balance by freeing her circulation and improving her oxygen intake.

# In Your Healing Space

We are going to free trapped energy by stimulating the flow of healing thoughts. First we will liberate the places where vitality has become stuck. This is easily done in a bath. That way you can wash away the past while you soak.

# A Hot Apple Cider Vinegar Bath

To a hot bath add two pints of apple cider vinegar. Soak for twenty minutes. Repeat this three days consecutively. We use apple cider vinegar because both the apples and the sour energy of vinegar cleanse the body, especially the liver.

Imagine that the bathwater dissolves from your body and mind everyone you have ever met. Starting from the top of your head down to your toes, go through your entire body very slowly, allowing your breath to erase everything and everyone except your healing space. Take as long as you need to until you start to relax. Inhale gently and, as you exhale, relax from your hair down through the soles of your feet.

It may help you to visualize all parts of you relaxing. Each time you exhale, mentally repeat such words as "My hair is relaxed; my scalp is relaxed; my brain is empty; my brain is perfect; my face is relaxed; my face is perfect; my neck is relaxed; my shoulders are supple; my heart is calm; my sexual area is empty; my body is beautiful" and any other phrases that make you feel completely satisfied to be alone, free, and strong.

Some areas will be full of memories. Pause there and repeat your calming words to give yourself a chance to heal more deeply. The following mixture will make it possible for you to purify profoundly.

# A Purifying Mixture

This part is optional but effective for gaining mental clarity. You will combine a powerful homeopathic remedy with one drop of your own blood in order for your body and emotions to be purified from the deepest part of you. You will be able to begin your life and love again by emotionally cleansing negative relationships and experiences from the inside out.

Sterilize a sewing needle by putting it into a flame until it turns red hot. Prick the tip of your middle finger and squeeze it to get one drop of blood. I chose that point because an acupuncture point there lowers anxiety. Then safely dispose of the needle in a labeled envelope.

Put the drop of blood into a clean white teacup. Add spring water to fill the cup, and add one dose of homeopathic ignatia 30c. Sip this water during your cleansing bath. The homeopathic remedy will work without the addition of your blood, but it will work deeper with it. Even though the effects of homeopathic remedies wear off as they are absorbed, your best benefits will come from reflecting upon what it is that you need to cleanse. The healing liquid you have created, a drop of your essence and a trace of Saint Ignatius's bean, will take a healing vibration to your blood to act as a catalyst for deep positive change.

Homeopathic ignatia is used to clear grief, loss of love, and terrible personal conflicts. It works by freeing those feelings so that you feel renewed. You may temporarily experience sadness after taking the homeopathic ignatia. That is the relief of shedding an old self. You can repeat this process during your cleansing baths.

The medical practice of combining homeopathic remedies with our blood was begun in the 1950s by the German physician Hans-Heinrich Reckeweg. My suggestion varies with his standard procedure—the blood and homeopathic mixture is not injected into a patient. In his theory, the patient's blood becomes its own detoxifying agent. Although you imbibe the cleansing mixture orally, the healing benefits can be absorbed as all homeopathic remedies are absorbed into the bloodstream through blood vessels under the tongue.

One main difference in making such a remedy at home instead of passively being injected in an expensive clinic is that you can enjoy the privacy of your healing space. The great power of using such a potion comes in visualizing what is being cleansed while you take it.

## Visualization

While sipping the homeopathic ignatia mixture, imagine that its cleansing vibration is carried to your blood, bone marrow, brain, sexual organs, and then to all parts of you so that you are purified of grief, sorrow, loss, rage, frustration, regret, and self-doubt. Ignatia removes mental and spiritual poisons from the past and present.

Make sure to take as long as you need to heal your loss. One woman I know, who was going through a long, painful divorce, used homeopathic ignatia and cleansing baths daily for two weeks. At the end of that time, she reported that she felt whole again and confident about her future.

# A Healing Activity

After three or more days of cleansing, active participation in your healing can begin. Feeling empty and purified is not enough. You cannot make progress with problems or higher development simply by being empty. You need to refill yourself with love for humanity and nature. Those who love nature can become part of it, benefiting from its strength, longevity, and fruitfulness. Nature and spirit heal you because they are limitless. The simplest creature has the life force necessary to fulfill its destiny, and you are not a simple creature but a person capable of thought, feelings, and the capacity to love. Using those skills will heal you.

## A Tiny Yellow Flower

Pulsatilla is a tiny yellow flower used by Chinese herbal doctors to clear mucus waste and parasites from the colon. Homeopathic doctors use a trace of pulsatilla to clear the lungs of congestion. The homeopathic remedy reduces excess sadness and crying. It lifts our spirits when we feel stifled, unable to breathe. Do you have psychic parasites sucking your life force? Do you find it hard to breathe through thick phlegm? Do you feel sluggish, overcome by grief and cares?

Become the pulsatilla. Even a tiny flower can be powerful when well applied. You can become an instrument of healing. The yellow pulsatilla is an astringent, disinfectant plant. It clears obscured thinking and grief. Using insights based upon your experience, you can create more clarity and understanding in others. You can and must become, in some sense, a healer to be able to heal yourself.

If you feel stuffed up with white or grayish phlegm, use homeopathic pulsatilla 30c, taking five doses daily between meals. It will clear your congestion, improve your energy, and lift your spirit. It will help you clear away the debris of heartbreak. Then you can be free to help others. By helping them, you will gain strength you never thought you had.

# A Cool Strong Metal

Some people experience heartache differently because their pain is buried deep inside them. Instead of loss, they feel the heat of rage or anxiety. Smoking, poor diet, and life in the fast track often turn heartache into hard-driving mania. Inflammatory habits turn mucus congestion into a dry raspy cough. Then emotional pain is not experienced so much as a wet heaviness in the chest but as choking and a dry mouth.

If you have a dry cough, thirst, fever, rage, parched skin, and a red tongue, use homeopathic silver, argentum nit. 30c instead of pulsatilla. The cooling, moistening effects of silver will heal emotional wounds and give you the fresh endurance of youth. Silver is moistening; pulsatilla is drying. You will be able to sense which you need most. The remedy that balances you will immediately feel right. After having loosened your congestion for a while with argentum nit. 30c, you can use the pulsatilla 30c to clear it away.

# A Tibetan Cure

Now that you've simplified and purified your feelings and established the sort of homeopathic remedy that keeps you in balance, you can begin to work on your karma. It's a basic belief among spiritual people the world over that we improve our lives by helping others. A friend of mine once put it simply: "We have to deserve our happiness."

When I was in Lhasa in the mid-1980s, I walked the *parcour* circling the Jo Khang temple along with Tibetan worshipers. Many had come from a great distance. Some prostrated themselves at full length, which is the custom in Tibet. They told their one hundred eight beads and recited prayers as the perfume of juniper incense filled the air. I saw a woman with her two children and a pet sheep circling the temple along with the others.

It was a common belief in traditional Tibet that to spare the life of an animal usually consumed as food was a worthy action. It increased good karma. I have seen similar acts of generosity among Chinese and Thai

Buddhists. Outside most Thai temples, people gather to watch traditional dance and music concerts. Usually there are men who sell tiny bright-colored birds in cages. Thai Buddhists buy the birds, recite prayers over them, wishing them well, and then release them into the air. Such acts of kindness create a sense of harmony both for the person giving freedom and for the birds. Giving alms to the poor or medicine to the sick is also advised for improving karma. That way, Buddhists believe, we can avoid trouble in this lifetime and in the next. Generosity shows us the way to be loving.

Perform an act of loving kindness for a stranger. Buy a freshwater fish and free it, or feed street cats or birds. Give food or clothes to homeless people or leave your gift on the street for them to find. Every tree or plant that you care for gives more oxygen to the world. You will feel the healing influence of these acts of kindness more directly than by writing a check to a charity.

You will heal as you directly take care of those who need your help. As a healer, you can cure your own loneliness and grief. If you love someone who does not love you, if you want to help someone who is incapable of accepting it, help someone else, show your love to someone else. If someone has hurt you, try to express your feelings with art—write, paint, or express your feelings somehow. Then use your art to help others. Your kindness is the better part of healing.

# Herbal Heart Remedies

Asian heart tonics that correct irregular heartbeat or angina work by freeing trapped circulation in the chest. They create a sense of freedom and well-being because they allow your thoughts and feelings to flow. They reduce congestion and heaviness in the chest, while they restore emotional tranquillity. When you combine heart tonic herbs with others that calm the spirit and dissipate congestion, you enhance mental clarity.

A number of herbal combinations are sold to treat such problems as restlessness, insomnia, palpitations, chest pains, and poor memory. They can be taken regularly until you regain focus. You can easily order them by calling or faxing one of the distributors listed at the back of this book.

# Chinese Herbal Pills

Ding Xin Wan is a Chinese patent remedy usually recommended for insomnia, poor concentration, and mental restlessness. It contains a number of herbs that harmonize heart action and adrenal energy, our source of endurance. I can't think of anyone I ever met who was upset or heartbroken who was not also exhausted. Even if a person is hyperactive from insomnia or a manic episode, the imbalance comes from nervous exhaustion. Stress is tiring. This remedy supports vitality and mental clarity. The normal dosage is five pills three times daily between meals, but you will be able to sense if that is enough.

When we're upset we often reach out to others from our heart with worry or agitation. We become exhausted. Then we need to strengthen our vitality, courage, and mental tranquillity. Ding Xin Wan is not a mind sedative but a blend of heart-balancing herbs. Also add a pinch of saffron to mint tea.

Xiao Yao Wan, a Chinese digestion remedy normally recommended for bloating, hypoglycemia, chest pain, or a lump-in-the-throat feeling, is useful for mental clarity and depression because it strengthens your emotional center. It makes you feel at home in your body. Your digestion will become smoother and your energy more regular if you take such digestive remedies. For severe depression and spaciness from hypoglycemia, I recommend that you take 30 to 40 or more pills daily.

# Susan's Cheerful Heart Tea

My friend, Susan Lin, who with her brother, Frank, owns Lin Sisters Herb Shop at 4 Bowery in New York City, has developed several herbal powder remedies using high-quality Chinese herbs. Her Cheerful Heart tea treats wakefulness, excess crying, chest aches, and depression. It contains herbs that build energy and reduce depression by strengthening the heart. Although the prescription varies according to individual needs, the major herbs used are most often Siberian and panax ginseng, schizandra, peony, rosebuds, and acorus rhizome.

# Depression, Exhaustion, and Yeast Infections

I have met women involved in long-term illness or difficult divorces who become emotionally exhausted. Exasperated, scattered, and out of sorts, they cannot think clearly. Uprooted from routine and stable yet unhappy home situations, they feel lost and powerless.

If that is your situation, it will be comforting to address your physical symptoms, not just the emotional trauma. That way you will feel more secure in your body, your power place.

If you have indigestion or poor circulation, you will feel pressure in the chest and gurgling in the abdomen. Often this can be assuaged by taking a digestive remedy along with one for yeast.

You do not have to have a "yeast infection" with burning yellowish vaginal discharge to have a yeast problem. Candida attacks those weakened by excesses in diet, insomnia, illness, surgery, and emotional stress. If you feel spacey and crave sweets or rich foods, it's likely that you have candida. See page 155 for information on how to cure a yeast problem with Australian Tea Tree Oil and homeopathic belladonna 30c. You can take both remedies between meals and follow meals with a digestive remedy such as Xiao Yao Wan. That Chinese patent remedy is especially effective in treating the vague foggy feeling that comes with hunger and weakness.

Saint John's wort capsules are recommended for depression. Although the herb is an antioxidant that improves brain blood circulation, it also has other effects. You will feel lighter and brighter after taking Saint John's wort because it helps digestion and breathing by clearing the sticky, heavy feeling of excess mucus. It is the anti-mucus aspect, the astringent quality, of the herb that improves oxygen intake in the body. With more oxygen, we think more clearly and feel stronger.

Other cures for low blood oxygen also clear mucus and fatty wastes. They include kava kava, a pepper, and three rejuvenating homeopathic tissue salts: kali. mur. and kali. sulph. (two forms of potassium), and nat. sulph. (a form of sodium that cleanses the liver). Add one dose of each homeopathic remedy to your morning tea for better breathing and digestion all day.

## Rosebuds in Your Tea

Chinese doctors treat depression by soothing the heart. Often their herbal formulas are complicated. One simple remedy is very easy to use at home. Add a handful of dried Chinese red rosebuds to your tea to lift the tight feeling from your chest. A favorite Chinese tea to use is called Po Nee, but oolong teas are also good. The perfume of the flowers is bittersweet, like love. Their quality is cooling, refreshing, and soothing, like a good vacation.

# Spiritual Apathy and Executive Burnout

Executives burn out in stages. Their backs ache, their pulses become weak, and their faces lose the glow of energy. As their heartbeat becomes irregular, they may compensate by reaching for rich foods or other addictions. That starts the roller coaster of fatigue, addictions, exhaustion, apathy, and self-recrimination. Stop the ride and get off the treadmill by adding these herbs to your life.

## Heart Weakness and Cholesterol

Hawthorn berries and green tea both come in capsules. They reduce harmful cholesterol and strengthen the heart. Take one capsule after meals if your heart feels shaky, slow, or irregular. Their quality is bitter-sour—just what you need to reduce fatty deposits in blood vessels. Dan Shen Wan, folic acid, and vitamin $B_6$ can also protect you. It is wise to follow the basic weight loss diet recommended in Chapter 9 and the advice from Chapter 8 to keep your energy high and reduce stress. It's more important than a big insurance policy.

## Chronic Diarrhea and Colitis

Do you ever find yourself thinking, "I can't take any more of this shit"? Do you also suffer from chronic diarrhea? Language never lies. My friends with colitis are all perfectionists. There is a Chinese remedy for weakness and habitual watery diarrhea caused by excess worry, weak digestion, and fatigue.

Bu Zhong Yi Qi Wan contains astragalus, licorice root, tang kuei, cimicifuga rhizome, codonopsis (false ginseng), atractylodes, citrus peel, bupleurum root, jujube (red date), fruit, and ginger. Its flavors are pungent, sour, and sweet. More than a digestive remedy that treats abdominal bloating, pain, and gas, it lifts prolapsed internal energy to treat hemorrhoids, varicose veins, and hernia. This combination is also useful for fatigue-related uterine bleeding and habitual miscarriage.

Do not use Bu Zhong Yi Qi Wan, a warming tonic, if you have a headache, fever, or a dry, reddish tongue, all of which indicate inflammation. The best remedy for hemorrhoids, varicose veins, and poor digestion for someone with ulcers or internal burning (a dry red tongue) is aloe vera gel. Add up to one-half cup daily to apple juice. If it gives you diarrhea, use less aloe and add twenty drops of gentian extract.

Gentian, most conveniently used in extract form, treats chronic diarrhea, shortness of breath, and depression related to poor digestion. Add ten to fifteen drops of this bitter after-dinner digestive to a little water. It helps reduce stomach irritation while it clears your thinking by improving digestion. Angostura Aromatic Bitters from the supermarket contains gentian and vegetable flavoring.

# In Your Healing Space

This chapter has shown you ways to clear depression and cloudy thinking as well as ways to soothe your heart and mend hurt feelings. Homeopathic remedies such as pulsatilla 30c and a combination of homeopathic potassium and sodium (page 63) are useful for clearing mucus and fat. Mucus is the sticky glue that keeps you down. It dampens vitality and muddles thinking because it slows metabolism and indirectly disrupts blood sugar balance.

Heart remedies such as hawthorn taken after meals or Ding Xin Wan at bedtime can help keep your heart in balance and working smoothly.

They will reduce physical pain. What you need is a way to bring your best energizing remedies together in a meaningful way in order to clear the air of evil influences, bad luck, poor karma, or dumb mistakes. I have met some lovely people who, because of circumstances beyond their control, seem to wear a label on their forehead that reads: "I'm a victim. Hit me."

---

## ❦ Heal Your Heart ❦

*H*ere is a guide for you to tear out and post somewhere at home and work. Listen to your words. They never lie.

*Indigestion/Hypoglycemia*

| | |
|---|---|
| "I'm fed up." | Xiao Yao Wan or |
| "I can't take any more of this garbage." | ginger, mint, cardamom tea |
| "They (it) make(s) me sick." | homeopathic nux vomica 30c |
| "I can't take it anymore." | |

*Mental and Physical Trauma and Long-Term Abuse*

| | |
|---|---|
| "You tear me apart." | Yunnan Paiyao or |
| "I feel beaten." | homeopathic arnica 30c |
| "You kill me!" | |

*Revenge Feelings*

| | |
|---|---|
| "I'm going to get you!" | Lung Tan Xie Gan Wan or |
| "I hate you!" | 20 drops skullcap extract |
| "You're a pain in the neck!" | |

*Exhaustion with Diarrhea*

| | |
|---|---|
| "I can't take any more of this shit!" | 20 drops gentian extract or homeopathic arsenicum 30c |
| "I am losing my guts!" | |

*Depression*

| | |
|---|---|
| "It's hopeless." | homeopathic pulsatilla 30c |
| "I am overcome." | or nat. mur. 30c |

# No More Abuse

Sometimes we don't have the energy or courage to protect ourselves from harmful situations. You may be stuck between a rock and a hard place, unable to free yourself. It pays to build physical stamina and mental clarity so that you can see your way out of the situation somehow. Both will improve with the following routine, which enhances breathing and circulation. Before you start, consider this advice.

People who lie down in front of moving trains get hurt. You may be part of someone else's abuse scenario. Protect yourself if you are closely associated with someone who is substance- or alcohol-dependent, insane, or abusive. If necessary do not answer the phone and get police protection. It does no good whatsoever to play victim. Make a separate life for yourself. You cannot live someone else's life. You may be a heroic person trying to do the impossible, but your partner-in-abuse must find his or her own way. You may have learned a lot of survival skills. You may have become used to living on the edge of danger. But you will be surprised at how well you will feel if you change your diet, use a few herbs, and then, as you become stronger, find a way to help the weak or impoverished.

# Protect Yourself

You can create a protective shield with herbs. Certain adrenal tonics such as Sexoton build vitality and confidence. Here is another way: put one drop of pure essential clove or bay oil three inches below your navel. Acupuncture points there deepen your breath to strengthen and relax you. Both oils are useful for depression. Clove is stimulating, useful for wheezing asthma and low energy. Bay is calming and enhances courage and centeredness. Wear your shield under your clothes. These warming oils will fortify and ground you. If you are overheated, they may make you feel uncomfortable. In that case, also add ten drops of skullcap extract to one cup of water and drink it anytime for headache, dizziness, and insomnia.

# Clear the Air

Here is a healing practice useful anytime you want to start over from scratch and build good luck. It increases oxygen intake so that your brain, heart, and defense systems work better.

All day long alternate doses of homeopathic ferrum phosphate 6x (iron) with kali. sulphate 6x (potassium). Each hour take one or the other. Together they gradually increase oxygen in the cells. Add one-quarter to one-half cup aloe gel to water and drink it throughout the day.

If you have been physically or psychically injured, take two capsules of Yunnan Paiyao after meals. See page 94 for information on this Chinese remedy for bruising and pain. It also works on an emotional level when you've been battered. It breaks apart holding and protecting patterns that make you withdraw into yourself to hide. Yunnan Paiyao eases your feelings of being beaten up.

Continue with this herbal regime for as many days as you need. Focus your attention on a photograph or a painting of an older person or an ideal energy that you want to become. Invite that positive energy into your healing space.

## Keys

Insomnia and agitation: Ding Xin Wan; valerian; gotu kola and
    Siberian ginseng capsules
Panic: homeopathic aconite 30c
Weepiness and excess mucus: homeopathic pulsatilla 30c
Exhaustion, fear of the future: homeopathic gelsemium 30c
Shock, grief, loss, no weeping: homeopathic ignatia 30c
Trauma: Yunnan Paiyao, homeopathu arnica 30c

Links: Also see Chapters 3, 8 (winter and Cancer: Extra-Strong Prevention, page 131), 13, 14, 15, 17

# CHAPTER 17

# You and the Cosmos

*Find the healing space within you.*

*Your Goal:* **To harmonize your biorhythms, simplify your life, and reduce stress.**

*Materials:* **Candles, plants, pet crickets or birds; beautiful sights, sounds, and aromas from nature, including incense and essential oils. Optional: musical instruments and drawing materials. A quote from Albert Einstein,** *The World as I See It,* **1931: "The trite objects of human efforts—possessions, outward successes, luxury—have always seemed to me contemptible."**

Aging is whatever makes you feel older, weaker, less engaging, or less active than you would like to be. In this chapter we will come to terms with ourselves as beings on a planet, living during a certain time and in a certain place. What makes you feel old? That is different from asking what hurts or needs improvement. It comes down to understanding who you are in terms of who you want to become. You can address the issue by engaging your relationship to earth's energies—color, sound, sight, fragrance—the sensual bath that envelops and protects you.

All the theories about aging mean little unless we can improve the quality of our life. Delaying cell reproduction in test tubes and modifying chromosomes in laboratories will not help. Instead, we need to temporarily stop our normal habits and take the time to feel more alive than our usual hectic pace allows. We will alter our normal biorhythms for a few days to find our way back to an older way of being in the cosmos. Doing this can awaken a deeper well of inspiration.

First, we must carefully eliminate outside noise and then watch what rises to the surface of consciousness. Here's an outline of what we will be doing. I'll explain each section in detail as we come to it.

# Harmonize Your Biorhythms with Nature

Choose a weekend or a few days during the full moon, a birthday, or whenever you need to rest. Invite friends to join you, or stay alone in your healing space at home:

> Turn off electric lights and gadgets, phones, computers, and televisions. Use candles.
>
> Using healing sights, sounds, and fragrances, create an inner balance according to a Chinese meridian clock.
>
> Balance your life force vitality in relation to the universe.
>
> Observe natural biorhythms, both day and night.
>
> Choose herbs and foods from among the lists I have provided.
>
> Use movements, baths, and massage to tone and relax.
>
> Do simple centering activities—drawing, making something.
>
> Share your joy with someone; care for a plant, pet, or person.
>
> Remember your heroes and heroines.
>
> Take a Tibetan Precious pill.
>
> Give something away—food, clothes, money, free work.

# There's a Time for You

Most Americans spend their energy looking at computer and television screens, eating junk on the run or foods zapped in microwaves, driving to and from work, arguing when they get there, and worrying. Have you tried the latest health fad for weight loss or depression? Do you recognize that there is a relationship between your lifestyle and your health?

Now's your chance to change things. Let's go back to the cave for a while. There's no television or refrigerator, but neither is there a time clock or a stock market. As a cave dweller, you can relax because things are rather simple. That's what this chapter is about—simplifying your life and improving your health.

We are going to retreat from modern life. Decide where and when to do this. A weekend will work as long as you change your schedule completely. We want to realign with nature's rhythms, not the city's or your family's. This vacation is just for you. If you do decide to invite a friend or two, please make sure they're willing to follow my directions back to the primeval forest. After you come out on the other end, you'll feel renewed with a savage vitality. To achieve this, you have to forget everything you've learned about being corporate or chic.

## Shut Out the Noise

Redecorate your healing space. Or better yet, transform an entire room in your home into a cave. Remove any lamps and anything that must be plugged in. Drape the walls, pictures, and mirrors with sheets or large pieces of green or brown cloth, or choose a print from nature. Burn incense that reeks of the woods or ocean. Create a place where you want to retreat to.

I like bringing in potted flowers. Once I had several birds in a cage, crickets in a shoe box, fish in a bowl, a tree frog, and a tiny pet snake in a terrarium. It was wonderful living in the country surrounded by its gentle sounds. For your weekend retreat, at least buy some crickets from a pet store. Keep them in a cage away from extreme temperatures. They eat raw apple.

When you have nature as your home, life rhythms can slow to a comfortable pace. Once on such a retreat, for days at a time, I threw open the shades, went to sleep early with the birds, and let them wake me at dawn. It was invigorating. I became able to trust New York City outside my window because of my country retreat inside. Even if you live in the country, you'll find it relaxing simply to turn off your connections with modern life.

# The Art of Balance—the Chinese Meridian Clock

Centuries ago while ancient philosophers were inventing the rules of acupuncture and Chinese medicine by observing nature, they realized that life proceeds in a rather predictable manner: our vitality ebbs and flows as if following the hours of an invisible clock. They correlated the workings of our body with the time of day or night. That gave them an idea of how to regulate our life force most efficiently.

Much later, modern research came up with the idea of biorhythms, but the Western notion of biorhythms lacks something essential, something profoundly healing. That is the notion of an energy body, the fundamental anatomy and physiology of traditional Asian medicine. Body processes are repeated with regularity. In other words, we have natural energetic internal rhythms.

It's very useful to know *which* of our various activities such as breathing, digesting, maintaining a steady heartbeat, and lovemaking are weaker or stronger at certain times of day based on those energy rhythms. We can learn the optimum time for all such activities by paying attention to the ancient Chinese meridian clock. I'll explain how we can also use this information for self-diagnosis and treatment.

Please glance at the following summary of the Chinese theory of cosmology, indicating the hours of the day and night and their relationship to internal organs and acupuncture meridians. This is the basis of classical Chinese biorhythms. Then read how I have applied that knowledge in order to guide us.

# A Schema of Classical Chinese Cosmology

| Hours | Organs, Meridians | Function | Herbs, Minerals |
|---|---|---|---|
| 7:00 A.M.–9:00 A.M. | Stomach, spleen | Digestion, elimination | Cleansing herbs, zinc |
| 9:00 A.M.–Noon | Heart | Circulation | Heart tonics, manganese |
| 12:00 P.M.–2:00 P.M. | Small intestine | Absorption, mental clarity | Warming, grounding digestives |
| 2:00 P.M.–5:00 P.M. | Bladder, adrenals | Expansive vitality, courage | Adrenal tonics, silver |
| 5:00 P.M.–7:00 P.M. | Kidneys | Hearing, sexual, memory, mental clarity, hormonal balance, immunity | Blood, energy herbs, gold |
| 7:00 P.M.–9:00 P.M. | "Triple heater" | Autoregulation, temperature | Balancing herbs |
| 9:00 P.M.–1:00 A.M. | Liver | Vision, detoxification, drive, muscle coordination, decisiveness | Blood cleansers and tonics, manganese |
| 1:00 A.M.–4:00 A.M. | Gallbladder | Digestion, determination | Anti-stone, anticholesterol herbs |
| 4:00 A.M.–7:00 A.M. | Lungs | Energy, breath, self-preservation | Mucus-clearing antibiotic herbs |

# How to Use Chinese Cosmology

The original classical Chinese hour clock contains information on the hours and their relationship to internal organs and meridians. To this I have added the functions of the internal organs according to classical Chinese medicine, and I've also provided some herbal suggestions. The herbs and minerals I recommend might be used to strengthen weak or damaged internal organs throughout the entire day. This will take some explaining. I shall be brief because I have specific recommendations for your at-home retreat. It comes down to how to organize your day. I offer a specific example on the following page. Feel free to use any diet recommendations or visualizations from other chapters.

Mornings—detoxify; stimulate digestion and circulation

Afternoons—build energy

Evenings—build blood, heal nerves and brain

Since morning energy is most conducive to digestion, cleansing, and circulation, it is wise to stress those types of herbs, foods, and activities. Choose from among pungent stimulant herbs and spices such as ginger, pepper, radish, and hot green or oolong teas. Add a drop of Australian Tea Tree Oil to a cup of tea to clear your senses. You can enhance digestion and energy by doing movements designed to free stuck vitality and digestive bile: stretching, walking, and deep breathing are a wonderful way to start the day. (See the slimming exercises from Chapter 10.)

Take time during midday hours to collect your thoughts and aspirations. Using herbs such as gotu kola or ginkgo to promote mental clarity and memory between meals will improve your energy and mood all day. Build sexual vitality during the late afternoon by adding one-quarter teaspoon of ashwagandha to hot water as a tea.

Use the evening hours to rejuvenate nerves and emotions. Blood tonics such as he shou wu, nerve tonics such as Siberian ginseng, and anti-inflammatory herbs such as American ginseng are useful for feverish conditions and rejuvenation.

# The Hour Clock and Diagnosis

You can also use Chinese cosmology as an aid to diagnosis. If you notice that your sparkle fades at the same time each day, it's very likely that the associated organ system is weakened by fatigue, overwork, or illness.

If you can't wake up in the morning, for example, try eating a lighter meal at night. Follow the evening meal with digestive herbs and an overnight laxative—perhaps one or two cascara sagrada capsules—at bedtime. This bitter stimulant laxative works roughly eight hours after you take it. Hot green or other laxative teas will get you moving in the morning. Doing stretches and massaging the stomach, legs, and feet while still in bed will also work.

If you can't stay awake between 3:00 P.M. and 5:00 P.M., or if your sexual vigor is low, it's likely that your adrenals are exhausted. You ought to use appropriate adrenal tonics such as damiana or ashwagandha. The advantage in using a healing herb instead of another cup of coffee at that time is that herbal tonics support rather than exhaust your energy.

After you become acquainted with Chinese time, you may revamp your day to utilize the hours to best advantage. Here's one retreat day:

---

# Organize Your Retreat: A Daily Example

| | |
|---|---|
| Dawn–7:00 A.M. | Up with the birds, hot cleansing tea, yoga stretches, tai chi, or a walk, deep breathing, skin brush, shower or bath with soda and salt. |
| 7:00–9:00 A.M. | Observe tongue, choose foods and herbs for the day. Breakfast: digestion, energy-building, anti-mucus, and anticholesterol herbs; hot digestive, cleansing tea and heart stimulant herbs—e.g., green tea, dandelion, hawthorn, ginger, cardamom, radish, Omega 3 oil, and calcium-source fish. |

| 12:00 noon–2:00 P.M. | Lunch: Hot tea with ginger and one pinch nutmeg for digestion and absorption; gotu kola capsules for centering and mental clarity; simple centering activity, remembered heroes or visualization, set things straight— letters, gifts, calls, make plans for next day, week. |
| 3:00–5:00 P.M. | Build vitality with breathing and movement, weight loss stretches, and kidney-adrenal (sexual) herbal tonics. |
| 5:00–7:00 P.M. | Eat a light dinner. |
| 7:00–9:00 P.M. | Social, sensual, sexual activities, including healing baths, hormonal massage (page 231); and visualizations for healing the past (see Chapters 14 and 16). |
| 9:00–10:00 P.M. | Blood- and moisture-building herbs, rest nerves (he shou wu, Siberian ginseng, gotu kola). Early to bed. |

# Special Herbs and Foods

As I mentioned, you should practice the individual diet and herbal recommendations that work best for you from previous chapters. In general it is best to use a cleansing or energy-focusing diet such as the basic one described on page 146, including fruits, vegetables, tofu, or fish and green tea.

This retreat may become an excellent opportunity to focus on one special problem. For diet and herbal remedies you can incorporate into your retreat, please turn to the following pages:

Arthritis, pages 61, 84, 85

Cancer, pages 131–135, 98–100

Depression, pages 266–269

Heart trouble and high cholesterol, Chapter 9

Low sexual energy and enthusiasm, pages 226–229

Weight loss, Chapters 9 and 10

Wrinkles and other beauty issues, pages 180–183

Do you want to have your retreat as a reward for hard work or as a comfort to ease stress? Here's a lovely rejuvenating massage and bath.

# Bath, Visualization, and Massage

Throughout this book I have provided special baths for balancing energy. I have described a teapot clean bath using soda and salt and a special vinegar soak designed to purify the liver. I like to add visualizations along with the bath because they provide an opportunity to focus thoughts and feelings. Now we'll enjoy a back-to-nature bath.

Running water in the wild is thrilling to see. It's energizing to be near a stream or river. Our vitality is enhanced by the movement. This recipe of aromatic herbs can be added to your bath to stimulate a similar pleasure.

## Herbal Jump-Start Bath

**¼ cup dried rosemary or 1 big handful fresh rosemary**

**¼ cup dried sage leaves or ⅛ cup fresh sage leaves**

**¼ cup dried thyme or ⅛ cup fresh thyme**

**¼ cup mint or 1 big handful fresh mint**

**1 quart water**

Bring all of the ingredients to a simmer and immediately turn off the heat. Steam your face for five minutes with the aromatic herbal brew, then strain the liquid into a tub of warm water. Soak for fifteen minutes. You might also give yourself the energizing massage described below. Follow this bath with a cool shower.

You might make a sachet of the above spicy herbs by putting one-quarter cup of each into a pillow made from a discarded silk stocking.

The fragrance will energize your bed or any other place you decide to put the pillow.

Rosemary stimulates the heart and the adrenal glands. As such it is a powerful energy stimulant and aphrodisiac. Sage also stimulates the whole body. Thyme increases breathing, and mint speeds digestion. All in all, this bath and sachet will boost your late afternoon energy. Use these herbs anytime you want to banish the blues.

# Visualization

This visualization is very simple. You have already done most of the preparation by redecorating your healing space in order to retreat into nature. Now visualize in full detail your natural surroundings.

Is it a setting you know from childhood or from vacations?

Is it a place you desire to visit for the first time?

What are the natural sights and sounds around you?

What do you want to do there now?

See the original you there, sans illness, problems, or fatigue.

What does your original self want to do in this natural setting?

What can your original self teach you about this place?

What can you learn here from your original self?

Relax and enjoy this corner of nature. Be there with your original self.

# An Energizing Massage

Massage can be soothing, relaxing, or sensually stimulating. This massage is designed to untie physical and emotional knots. Stuck circulation can turn into lumps and bumps in your abdomen, back, or legs. By dissolving those knots, you free the way for vitality, youth, and emotional growth.

The following massage is based on acupuncture principles. For professionals, I have listed important points to stress. (See luo points on page 285.) Everyone will greatly benefit from massaging these areas because they are pockets of trapped energy.

You can do this massage for a few minutes or for up to an hour. It can be done with or without oil. If you use oil, add essential lavender oil to olive oil. Lavender unlocks energy blocks, and olive oil is healthy no matter how you absorb it.

Use strong counterclockwise circular movements with the palms of your hands and the flat tips of your fingers. Do not poke or pinch. Make sure the room temperature and your hands are warm. Work from the head down toward the feet, first on the front of the body, then the back. If you are giving the massage to someone else, make sure to coordinate your breath with that person's. Breathe slowly together for five minutes before you begin. You can also do this massage in the stimulating bath.

# Let Yourself Flow

Working slowly and pressing in a deep but comfortable manner, these are the areas to massage:

Scratch head, massage neck, tops of shoulders, roll the
  shoulders
Massage chest, down inner arm to palms
Counterclockwise circles over heart and each breast
Massage down outer arm, fingers
Stretch torso out in all directions, reaching with arms and legs
Circular clockwise massage on abdomen
Stand, stretch forward, reach toward opposite wall, and relax
  down
On all fours, bend spine up and down like a cat
Curl into a ball, then release
Roll and twist hips side to side on floor
Repeat circular massage on abdomen
Massage down inner thighs, and inner calves, massage away all
  bumps counterclockwise
Continue down to inner ankle and bottoms of feet, roll ankles
Stretch out lengthwise in both directions, then release
Massage down tops of legs and around knees and outside legs

Continue to outer ankle crease and entire top of foot
Lie flat, touch lower back to floor, and then relax completely

---

To my massage therapy, acupuncture, and chiropractic friends: When you do this massage, include these Xi (cleft) points according to the time of day or if there are stagnation symptoms with the related organs. They are points on acupuncture meridians used to move stuck energy in the meridian or area it passes through. See *Essentials of Chinese Acupuncture* or other such text for point locations. I've listed the number and Chinese name:

Spleen 8, diji
Heart 6, yinxi
Pericardium 4, ximen
Lung 6, kongzui                    **Morning**
Inner wrist toward elbow
Large intestine 7, wenliu

Sanjiao triple heater 7, huizong
Small intestine 6, yanglao          **Noon**
Outer wrist up to outer elbow

Stomach 34, liangqiu
Gallbladder 36, waiqiu
Urinary bladder 63, jinmen
Top and front of knee, down
    outside leg to outside ankle
Then top of feet                    **Afternoon**
Liver 6, foot-zhongdu
Kidney 5, shuiquan
Inside calf, down to ankle, rub out all bumps
Then bottoms of feet

# A Simple Centering Activity

Repeating an ordinary task, while focusing all your attention on it, can quiet the mind. It is the basis of Zen meditation. From that quiet mind, positive change can arise. Watching a repeated activity is also pleasing. In one of San Francisco's great restaurants, I once witnessed a moving meditation:

*I have come to watch the graceful art of the sushi man. Every night he performs a show. He does not see me watching him from across the room. He wields a large pointed knife, cutting exactly the same angle, exactly the same width. Tilting his head slightly, he moves as in a dance with each slice. He has become a part of his brother fish, sees the river where the fish swam. I've come tonight to admire the art of the sushi man, his quiet respect for his skill and his dedication to his work.*

Choose a simple centering exercise for yourself. It may be copying a drawing over many times until it's perfect, or playing a musical scale. Choose something you do not ordinarily do. Find a part of you that you do not know. Practice part of an activity you would like to learn. For example, if you always wanted to play the flute, repeat only one note until you love the sound, until that one note becomes music.

To focus on your centering activity, use these herbs that quiet and direct the mind inward: gotu kola and Wuchaseng, a liquid form of Siberian ginseng available in Chinatown shops or by mail order. Take two capsules of gotu kola and one-half teaspoon of liquid extract. If you are so exhausted that this combination puts you to sleep, go ahead; you deserve the rest. When you are ready for the centering exercise again, use only the gotu kola.

## Remembered Heroes and Heroines

While taking a break from writing this chapter, I turned on the television with no special intention. It was Dr. Martin Luther King, Jr. giving the last minutes of his "I have a dream" speech on the steps of the Lincoln Memorial. I sobbed to see and hear him again, knowing that I love him more now than I did thirty years ago. The camera froze an instant of inspiration and hope that looked forward with courage. America has not fully met the challenge of his dream.

He was my hero, and I sorely felt the weight of my respect for him. There were fights at school and at the dinner table until I was finally forbidden to discuss religion, politics, or race. I knew only a few people of color when I was in high school in Albuquerque, but I knew segregation was wrong. Once when someone mocked, "Are you for 'em or agin 'em?"

I said, "For 'em." That opened the door to my accepting blacks, Jews, gays, and all others who were different, not family, especially myself. Seeing Dr. King again reminded me of myself as a kid, passionately committed to living life my way.

> Who were your heroes and heroines when you were young?
>
> Have you changed your ideas about them? Or your ideals?
>
> Have you been able to work toward those ideals?
>
> How can you help to accomplish them in some way?

## Sharing Joy

Sometime during your nature retreat, take time to contact those you have been too busy to acknowledge. Write letters or do some artwork. Remember, during the retreat lights are out by 9:00 P.M.

If you want to improve your karma, take care of unfinished business with letters of forgiveness, approval, or anything that brings the relationship to a higher level. You may also want to share your renewed sense of well-being by offering to help someone.

Our retreat does not end in the cave where we started. Withdrawing to nature gives a taste of freedom from exhaustion and care. You will be able to return to the world a different person, ready to tackle your work and worries until the next vacation in your cave. You have learned some valuable ways to get in touch with yourself. You have created a new self, based on the burned-out dreams of the original you. Your beauty and vitality can grow as you involve your new self in acts of loving kindness.

## Keys

Anxiety: Wuchaseng (Chinese extract of Siberian ginseng), Ding Xin Wan pills

Poor memory, nervousness: gotu kola capsules

**Links:** Also see Chapters 13, 14

# Parting Words

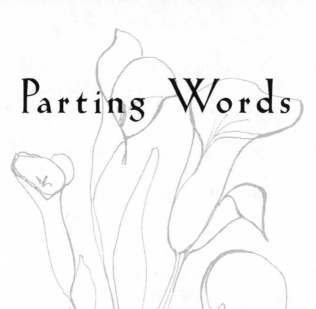

The summer's work is done. Our pussycats have become fat and jolly playing on the banister of our large Vermont house. Michael wrote his book on the famous French woman explorer of Tibet, calling it *The Secret Lives of Alexandra David-Neel*. Soon we'll return to New York, where I'll teach corporate rejuvenation workshops and make health videos.

I have enjoyed talking with you while writing this book. It has been fun concocting and trying my rejuvenation recipes on myself and friends. I have attained my ideal weight with slimming diets and herbs. I eliminated my carpal tunnel syndrome in less than one month with herbs, raw juices, and the special acupuncture massage described in Chapter 6.

As usual during the summer, I've used Chinese anticancer herbs, this time melting several lumps. I hope you have enjoyed adding my suggestions, recipes, and health practices to your personal quest for rejuvenation. Benefits gained from such self-analysis, prevention, and healing affect every aspect of your life.

A newspaper columnist once asked me how I manage to look so young. She had described me as looking like a thirty-year-old Swedish ski instructor even though I'm considerably older. I replied, "I'm in love, I use herbs, and I do what I can to help others." Natural remedies have given me the freedom to expect the best from myself—the best energy, mental clarity, beauty, and longevity possible for me. Because of that, I feel free from the threat of illness and aging.

Another Vermont summer has come and gone. We've found beautiful fruits and vegetables at farmers' markets, attended concerts, enjoyed church suppers, and visited dear friends. We've watched the swamp change colors many times.

Now the goldenrod is turning amber. The stately white Queen Anne's lace is half closed with the setting sun. There is bright orange echinacea growing along the edge of the water. Pale blue columbine and red clover are here as a single surprising purple thistle catches the light. I don't see the heron, but I imagine him here. The swamp welcomes me with green arms, holding its breath while awaiting the crystalline winter.

Every season has its colors. This one is muted gold and amber-green. All life comes from and goes back to this swamp. It never dies, only changes. I take in the sound of crickets and the smell of grass turned to sweet hay as I become a part of this swamp. It becomes a part of my healing space. From the center of my heart in this healing place, I send you my love.

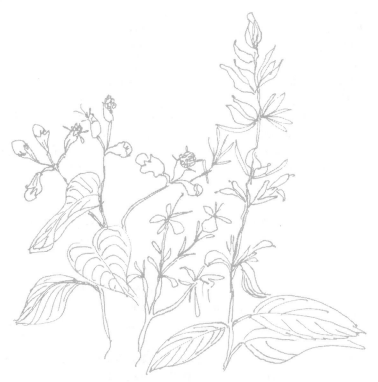

# Herbal Pronunciation Guide

Over the years my health clients have enjoyed trying to pronounce the names of the Asian herbs I have recommended for them. They rarely resemble English. There's an old joke about someone trying to learn German by repeating "donkey field mouse" in order to remember *danke viel mals* (thanks a lot). The following guide to Chinese, Latin, and Sanskrit herb names that appear in this book uses a similar approach with American syllables. It will familiarize you with a number of important Asian remedies.

**CAPS = for stressed syllables (if necessary)**
**(e) = pronounced deep in the throat as though burping**

**Ashwagandha:** Ahsh-wah GAHN dah

**Astragalus:** Ass-TRAG-gul-us

**Atractylodes:** Ah tract til lotus

**Bah Wei Di Huang Wan:** BAH way DEE whoo-ang wahn (aka Sexoton)

**Bupleurum:** Boo PLURR um

**Bu Zhong Yi Qi Wan:** Boo CHONG eee chee wahn

**Chih Ko and Curcuma:** Chick KOH and sircooma

**Chyavanprash:** CHAH vahn prahsh

**Dan Shen Wan:** DAHN shun wahn

**Ding Xin Wan:** DING shin wahn

**Gan Mao Ching:** GAHN maw ching

**Gan Mao Ling:** GAHN moh ling

**Gotu Kola:** Goh too COH la

**Gou ji tse:** Goh GEE z(e)

**Guan Jie Yan Wan:** Goo-ahn geh yahn wahn

**Jujube:** Joo JOO bay (hong zhao)

**Kang Gu Zeng Sheng Pian:** Kahng goo zung shung pee-n

**Lian Bai:** Lee-ann BUY

**Lien Chiao Pai Tu Pien:** LEE-N chee-aw BUY too pee-n

**Liu Wei Di Huang Wan:** Lee-oh WAY DEE whoo-ang wahn

**Lung Tan Xie Gan Wan:** LOONG tahn see-EH gahn wahn

**Rehmannia:** Rim MAH nee-ah

**Sexoton:** SEX oh tahn

**Sheshecao:** SH(E)-SS(E) tsah-oo

**Shilajet:** Shi LAH jeet

**Shou Wu Chih:** SOH ooo ch(e)

**Shou Wu Pien:** SOH ooo pee-n

**Strong Xiao Jin Tan:** Strong SEE-aw gen tahn

**Tang Kuei:** Tahng kway (or) Dohng kway

**Tienchi:** Tee-N-chee

**Wuchaseng:** OOO chah shan

**Xiao Yao Wan:** SEE-aw yee-AW wahn

**Yunnan Paiyao:** YOO-nahn BUY-yaw

**Zhi Bai Ba Wei Wan:** Z(e) buy BAH way wahn

# Herbal Access

Most of these companies will sell by mail order. If the distributor will not sell directly to you, have your neighborhood health food store order the product from them.

If you are unsure of the spelling or pronunciation of Asian herbs, photocopy a page from this book and mail or fax it to the distributors. For fun, also see the Herbal Pronunciation Guide.

## Ayurvedic Herbs

**ADH Health Products, Inc.**
215 N. Rte. 303
Congers, NY 10920
916-939-1860; 1-800-292-6002
Fax 916-939-1861

**Advanced Sports Nutrition**
Box 1277
Hood River, OR 97031
541-387-4500
Fax 541-387-4503

**Alchem International, Ltd.**
201 Empire Plaza
Mehrauli Gurgaon Rd.
Sultanpur, New Delhi
110 030 India
Fax 91-11-680-2102

**Al-Kemi**
3107 W. Colorado Ave. #277
Colorado Springs, CO 80904
719-685-5476
Fax 1-888-435-6618

**Ayurvedic Concepts**
6950 Portwest Dr., Suite 170
Houston, TX 77024
713-863-1622
Fax 713-863-1686

**Butala Emporium**
37-11 74th Street
Jackson Heights, NY 11372
718-899-5590
Fax 718-899-7889

**Gaia Herbs**
108 Island Ford Rd.
Brevard, NC 28712
704-884-4242
Fax 800-717-1722

**Zandu**
70, Gokhale Rd. S.
Dadar, Mumbai 400 025
India
Fax 91-22-437-5491
E-mail:
    Zanduho@giasbm01.vsnl.net.in
(Health Fit, Kesari Jivan [nutritional boost]; Mentoton [brain food]; Re-Juvin [ashwagandha supplement])

# Chinese Herbs

**APP Pharmacy**
197 Eighth Ave.
New York, NY 10011
212-691-9050; 1-800-227-1195
Fax 212-691-9052
(Asian herbal combinations and major
brands of Western herbs and vitamin
supplements)

**Crane Herb Company**
745 Falmouth Road
Marhpee, MA 02649
1-800-227-4118
Fax 508-539-2369

**Health Concerns**
8001 Caowell Dr.
Oakland, CA 94621
510-639-0280; 1-800-233-9355
Fax 510-639-9140
(Health Concerns, Seven Forests,
Zand, and Turtle Mountain; herbal
consultations)

**Kamwo Herb and Tea Company**
211 Grand Street
New York, NY 10013
212-966-6370
Fax 212-226-4717
E-mail: mailorder@kamwo.com

**Lin Sisters Herb Shop**
4 Bowery
New York, NY 10013
212-962-5417/0447
Fax 212-587-8826
(Bulk herbs, extracts, patent remedies, teas, herbal consultations)

**Shen Enterprises**
400 El Cerro Blvd., Suite 105
Danville, CA 94526
510-522-9888
Fax 510-460-5976
(Guang Ci Tang Concentrated Pills;
top-quality Chinese formulas manufactured in Shanghai)

# Organic Western Herbs, Extracts, and Bulk Herbs

**Amazon Herb Company**
725 North Aia, Suite C-115
Jupiter, FL 33477
561-575-7663
Fax 561-575-7935

**Arizona Natural Products**
8281 E. Evens Rd., Suite 104
Scottsdale, AZ 85260
602-991-4414
Fax 602-596-1628

**Bioriginal Food & Science Corp.**
#1 411 Downey Rd.
Saskatoon, SK S7J3Z5
Canada
306-975-1166
Fax 306-242-3829

**Bio-Selen Ltd.**
4 Baltimore St.
Petah-Tikva 49130
Israel
972-3-9264854
Fax 972-3-9248548

**Botanical Products Intl., Inc.**
Box 174
Hakalau, HI 96710
808-963-6771
Fax 808-963-6143

**Complete Nutritional Food Pty Ltd.**
24 Fremantle St.
Burleigh, Qld 4220
Australia
61-7-5522-1885/-6
Fax 61-7-5522-1887

## Japanese Natural Health Products

**Intelligent Choice, Inc.**
500 W. Harbor Dr. 1602
San Diego, CA 92101
1-888-252-PURE (7873)
Fax 619-702-3366
http://www.health1.com
(Konjac, chitosan, ashitaba, green tea, and LEM shitake capsules, Vegeta-gel [Jell-O], and Soft Natura konjac facial sponges)

**Yaohan**
333 South Alemeda St.
Los Angeles, CA 90017
213-687-6699
Fax 213-697-3405

## Bernard Jensen's Products and Books

**Bernard Jensen International**
24360 Old Wagon Road
Escondido, CA 92027
760-749-2727
Fax 760-749-1248
(Books)

**Bernard Jensen Products Company**
PO Box 8
Solana Beach, CA 92075
1-800-755-4027
Fax 619-755-2026
(Nutritional products)

## Homeopathic Remedies

**Boericke & Tafel**
2381 Circadian Way
Santa Rosa, CA 95407
707-571-8202
Fax 707-571-8237

**Boiron**
6 Campus Blvd., Bldg. A
Newton Sq., PA 19073
610-325-7464
Fax 610-324-7480

# Nutritional and Sports Supplements

**Amerifit**
166 Highland Park Dr.
Bloomfield, CT 06002
860-242-3476
Fax 860-286-8757

**Bio Dynamax**
6565 O'Dell Pl.
Boulder, CO 80301
303-530-2525
Fax 303-516-5235

**Biotech Corp.**
628 Hebron Ave., Bldg. 2, Suite 108
Glastonbury, CT 06033
860-633-8111
Fax 860-682-6863

**Tibetan Precious Pills**
write to:
Tibetan Medical Institute
Khara Danda Rd.
Dharamsala 176215
Dist. Kangra (H.P.) India
(Rinchen Mangjor Chenmo)

# Herbal Information Organizations

**American Botanical Council**
PO Box 201660
Austin, TX 78720-1660

**American Herbal Products Assoc.**
4733 Bethesda Ave., Suite 345
Bethesda, MD 20814
301-951-3207
Fax 301-951-3205

**American Holistic Health Assoc.**
Box 17400
Anaheim, CA 92817
714-779-6152
Fax 714-777-2917

# On-Line Health and Herbal Information

**Better Health Medical Network**
Health databases, chats, organizations,
    Healthwise Handbook
www.betterhealth.com

**Crane Herb Company on-line**
Health practitioner directory; manu-
    facturer and research information
info@craneherb.com

*Delicious!* **magazine on-line**
Also health and healing index, what's
    cookin'; natural search—a special-
    ized search engine exclusively for
    the natural products industry
www.delicious-online.com/ (See
    October 1997 for my article on
    women's herbs.)

**Healing Arts**
From Canada
www.healing-arts.com

**HealthLink**
On-line resources—database, dictionary, practitioners
www.healthlink.com

**Healthtouch**
Health resource directory
www.healthtouch.com

**Healthy Ideas**
Rodale Press's health magazine
www.healthyideas.com

**Herbal Information Center**
Order herbs and books on-line
www.koweb.com/herb/
herbmain.htm

**Institute for Traditional Medicine**
On-line article index for Chinese,
Tibetan, Ayurvedic, Thai, and
Native American medicine
www.europa.com/-itm

**The Mayo Clinic**
Research information on illnesses,
medical drugs, and herbal research
Mayo Health O@sis: www.mayo.edu

**Medline**
International herbal research abstracts
(use Latin botanical names)
www.infotrieve.com/healthworld
or
Healthworld Medline Search
www.healthworld.com/library/
search/medline.htm

**NEXUS**
Colorado's Holistic Journal
www.nexuspub.com

**Nutrition Science News**
A New Hope Natural Media publication for the health food store
industry
www.nutritionsciencenews.com

**Rocky Mountain Herbal Institute**
Chinese herbal education and
research
www.rmhiherbal.org

**Thrive**
Time Warner's health magazine
www.thriveonline.com

# Acknowledgments

I wish to thank Michael Foster, novelist, biographer, and philosopher, who has taught me that health and beauty can be accomplished only through living one's ideals.

The many fine hand-drawn herbal illustrations in this book are by my mother and illustrator, Letha Elizabeth Hadady of Albuquerque. As in *Asian Health Secrets,* her art is a beautiful teaching device. Also in Albuquerque, my lovely sister, Michelle, has been my trusted ally, and my brother, Eric Hadady, D.C., is my fitness adviser.

I am thrilled to have a foreword written by Dr. Bernard Jensen of Escondido, California—and the world. We met in the early 1980s during his seminar taught at the Omega Institute in upstate New York. His sweet disposition and profound insights concerning natural healing, human nature, and the state of modern health care made a lasting impression on me. A doyen of American alternative medicine, he has seen his art and craft turn from a profession at one time considered far-fetched if not illegal into one accepted by the mainstream and populated by gurus. Dr. Jensen has staunchly defended his right to treat illness with safe and sane natural cures. His courage, determination, spiritual radiance, and common sense are an inspiration to two generations of American healers. In radiant good health at age ninety, he writes books and travels throughout the country teaching seminars on natural health.

This book, like all my writing, has been a labor of love. To bring it into being, I have enlisted the help of friends. I especially want to thank Anna Abreu. I thank Ellen Geiger, my literary agent at Curtis Brown Ltd. in New York. My editor at Harmony Books, Shaye Areheart, has been a joy to work with. Her care has helped this book get my message across in a graceful, clear manner. My thanks also go to Dina Siciliano, Lauren Dong, Mary Schuck, and Barbara Balch at Harmony. My composer friend, Elma Meyer, has encouraged me and made suggestions for the book. My students at Sony Music Entertainment, the New York Botanical Gardens, and the New York Open Center have helped refine the rejuvenation programs. I would like to especially thank Paul Rush at the New York Open Center.

Designer Donna Karan and Jane Turker have exposed my healing work and books to a wide audience of press and magazine professionals.

I would also like to thank several magazine editors and media personalities who have furthered my work—Lynn Komlenic of *Natural Health and Fitness*, Dena Nishek at *Nutrition Science News*, Holly Levine at *Fitness*, Jane Larkworthy at *Jane*, Nicole Brechka of *Let's Live*, Denise Schipani of *Marie Claire*, Lois Joy Johnson and Jessica Goldman at *MORE*, and Judith Asphar and Vicki Carlyle at *Healthy Living*. I am happy to have been featured in the October 1997 issue of *Delicious!* magazine. Barbara Smith—NBC's B. Smith with Style—and her staff have been very helpful. Gary Null, alternative health's freedom fighter, has invited me many times to speak with him on radio. David and Linda Laskowski of WPON radio in Michigan, Rich Massabny of Arlington Cable Television, Stephan Mason of University of California Radio Network, David Essel, a syndicated radio personality and a walking advertisement for health and fitness, and, in San Francisco, Patrice Wynn, the spirited owner of Gaia Books, Josette King at Borders, and Lisa de Flaun at Book Passage, have all lent their enthusiastic support.

Several health professionals have kept me well. I give loving thanks to Nancy Hokensen of Titusville, New Jersey, a highly evolved acupuncturist healer. Dr. Lili Wu of Brooklyn has been my devoted Chinese doctor, and Susan Lin of Lin Sisters Herb Shop in New York, has been my herbalist and dear friend for many years. I thank the gentle Linda van Horn for her massage. I am indebted to Ilya Simakovski, D.C., of New York, whose excellent chiropractic care has made a difference in my work. I wish him luck in his writing projects. Skip Ishii, president of Intelligent Choice in San Diego, has educated me on the healing benefits of traditional Japanese health foods.

# Index

harmony with nature, 275
hawthorn, 42, 145, 147, 158,
    207, 224, 269, 270
headaches
    prevention plan for, 49
    remedies for, 117, 120, 124,
        125, 131, 239, 272
healing activity, 264–65
healing space, 15–20
    autumn in, 131
    creation of, 16–17
    emotional clearing in,
        125–26
    and five elements, 18–20
    freeing trapped energy in,
        261–64
    heart remedies in, 270
    hormonal massage in, 232
    incense in, 19
    lifting circulation and
        wrinkles in, 178
    plants in, 166
    as sanctuary, 256
    smaller version of, 17
    springtime in, 120–21
    summer in, 125–26
    viewing body shape in, 143
    virtual getaways in, 149–50,
        152–53, 159–60
    visualization in, 32, 114–15,
        256–58, 263
    winter in, 114–15
    within you, 274–87
    and work, 236
heart
    ankles and, 162–63
    broken, 259–73
    herbs for, 146, 179–80, 207,
        224, 266, 269
    keys, 273
    palpitations of, 207–8
Heart Tonic, Susan Lin's, 179–80
Heckart, Eileen, 238, 240
Herbal Jump-Start Bath, 282
Herba Oldenlandia Diffusa
    Beverage, 55
herbs
    anticancer, 99–100, 128
    antifever, 130, 132
    anti-fibroid, 38–39
    antiparasite, 103–4
    anti-phlegm, 53
    antiseptic, 146–47
    antitumor, 132, 133
    aphrodisiac, 128, 198, 227–28
    astringent, 146–47
    bitter, 146–47, 215–16
    for bloating, 151
    for circulation, 84–85, 179,
        228, 239
    cleansing, 46, 53, 146–47,
        162, 200, 215–16
    for cold and flu, 128
    cooling, 56, 59, 190–91,
        204, 211–12, 240

and cosmology, 278
diaphoretic, 180, 182
digestive, 151, 156, 169,
    222–23, 239
diuretic, 117, 158–59, 162,
    215
in face-lift, 180–84
for facial circulation, 71
for healthy intestinal bacteria,
    172–73
for the heart, 146, 179–80,
    207, 224, 266, 269
heating, 157, 188, 204, 211
hormone-balancing, 162
for immunity, 239
laxative, 147, 150–51, 215
for menopause, 188–90, 192
moistening, 42, 183,
    190–93, 239, 240
for pain relief, 171–72
quieting, 286
for rejuvenation, 239
and retreat, 281–82
for sexuality, 49, 111, 226,
    239
soothing, 118, 239
for soups, 110, 128, 131
for spring, 117, 118, 119
stimulating, 131, 157
for stress, 49, 113, 267
for summer, 123, 124
tonic, 95, 132, 204
for vitality, 110
weight-loss, 147, 158–59
for winter, 110, 111–12
herpes, 120
he shou wu, 112, 192, 216, 226
hijiki, 147, 199
hips, spot reduction for, 162–63
homeopathic remedies
    canceling the action of, 229
    when to take, 129
honey, 55
honey bee, homeopathic, 119
honeysuckle, 62, 123–24, 127,
    130, 181
hops, 113
hormonal creams, 194–95
hormonal massage, 231–34
horse chestnut capsules, 162
horse chestnut seed extract, 79
horseradish, 86
hot flashes, 125, 187–88, 215
hunger, and emotional binges,
    144–45
hypericum, 94
hypertension, 145
hypoglycemia, 113, 131, 209, 267

Ignatia, 229, 262–63
illness
    chronic, 256–57
    liver repair after, 216
    prevention of, see prevention
    recovery from, 91–104

immunity
    and chemotherapy, 99–100
    and energy, 213–14
    herbs for, 239
incense, 19, 120
indigestion
    from chemotherapy, 99
    and energy, 209
    prevention plan for, 48–49
    remedies for, 130, 151, 156,
        169, 209, 222–23, 239,
        250–51, 268
    and sex, 224
    teas for, 59, 114, 123
inflammatory conditions, 26
injury
    muscle pain from, 171–72
    recovery from, 91–104
    roots of, 256
insomnia, 112–14, 125, 128,
    207, 215, 267, 272
intestines
    and facial observation, 29
    healthy bacteria in, 172–73
    parasites in, 101–4
iron, homeopathic, 62, 113, 167,
    199

Japan, virtual trip to, 159–60
Jensen, Bernard, 248–49
jet lag, cure for, 237–38
joint pain, 49, 86, 117, 196,
    199
joints, rebuilding of, 148
juices, slimming, 157–58
jujube, 181, 182, 183
juniper, 158
juniper berries, 115, 117
junk-food addiction, 154–59

Kang Gu Zeng Sheng Pian, 196
karma, Tibetan cure for, 265–69
kava kava, 113, 147, 268
kelp, 147, 199
kidney-adrenal tonic, 196
kidney energy tonics, 213–14
kindness, 246
King, Martin Luther Jr., 286–87
knees, massage of, 174
kombu, 147, 237
Konjac, 159, 160

Lavender flowers, 131
lavender oil, 32, 178
laxatives, 147, 150–51, 161–62,
    215
lecithin, 117, 147
ledum (marsh tea), 94
leech, powdered, 133
legs
    Asparagus Legs Juice, 78–79
    herbs for, 172–73
    spot reduction for, 162–63
    tired, 78
    varicose veins of, 78–79

# ❧ ASIAN HEALTH SECRETS ❧
# Video

## *with Letha Hadady, D. Ac.*

Filmed on location in New York's Chinatown, the *Asian Health Secrets* video is based on Letha Hadady's best-selling book. In this entertaining and informative video, you will learn how to balance your energy, boost your immune system, and prevent and treat illnesses and common maladies by using the powerful diagnostic techniques and herbal remedies of Asian medicine.

The *Asian Health Secrets* video offers practical advice on how to use a variety of herbs, teas, extracts, and pills as safe and inexpensive alternatives or complements to Western treatments. Letha Hadady presents simple yet thorough diagnostic methods that will allow viewers to determine their daily herbal and dietary needs in order to promote total health and well-being. Hadady reveals ancient cures for a variety of ailments that were, for centuries, known only to Eastern healers.

"One of the nation's experts on Chinese remedies is leading a quiet ladylike revolution, bringing herbal remedies from the Far East into everyday use in American homes."

*San Francisco Chronicle-Examiner*

*ASIAN HEALTH SECRETS* Video • #76432 • 60 minutes • $19.98
To order, call 1-800-292-9001
or write:
MYSTIC FIRE VIDEO
P.O. Box 422, Dept. PRB
New York, NY 10012-0008
www.mysticfire.com
Add $4.95 for shipping and handling.
NY and CA residents add 8.25% sales tax.

# About the Author

L etha Hadady, D.Ac., is an herbalist and nationally certified acupuncturist. A graduate of the University of New Mexico, the University of Paris, and the Tri-State Institute for Traditional Chinese Medicine, she has continued her studies abroad at the Institute for Acupuncture and Meridians in Shanghai and the Institute for Tibetan Medicine in Dharamsala, India. An adjunct faculty member of the New York Botanical Gardens, she has worked with doctors of traditional Asian medicine in the United States and the Far East.

Her classes include her well-known walking tours of Asian herb markets given for such institutions as CBS, the New York Open Center, the Sierra Club, the Museum of Natural History, Columbia University, and New York Medical College.

She has conducted Personal Renewal workshops for clients such as Sony Music Entertainment, Staten Island University Hospital, and the New York Botanical Gardens. For information concerning these corporate rejuvenation workshops, please contact:

**Karma Unlimited, Inc.**
245 Eighth Avenue, Suite 364
New York, NY 10011
lethah@earthlink.net

Letha writes a bimonthly column on herbs for *Natural Health and Fitness* magazine. She is frequently featured in the media. Recently she has appeared as an herbal expert on CNN's *Burden of Proof.* Other recent appearances have been on NBC, CBS, America's Talking Network, the Food Channel, Lifetime, and NET. Radio interviews include the Associated Press, UPI, NPR, and hundreds of national and internationally syndicated stations, as well as on-line radio.

Letha was on the cover of *Delicious!* magazine and has been featured in *Jane, Let's Live, Healthy Living, Condé Naste Traveler, The New Yorker, Fitness, Marie Claire, More, Shape,* and *Allure. Newsday* has called Letha "the best-known blonde in Chinatown."